THE EASY ANTI-INFLAMMATORY DIET

Author
Mia Anderson

1

Table of contents

INTRODUCTION

"Inflammation" is tossed around a lot nowadays. There are numerous items that are promoted as being "anti-inflammatory" however, we should begin with the rudiments. What precisely is inflammation? Inflammation is the manner in which the body reacts to an aggravation. It very well may be a reaction to microbes, growths, infections, chemicals, and outer or inward wounds. That essentially implies that a healthy measure of inflammation is acceptable and can shield the body from annoyances. Be that as it may, similarly as with everything, an overabundance sum is rarely acceptable, and balance is vital.

What does it feel like when the body is over-burden with an overactive provocative reaction? Numerous people frequently feel depleted, hot, and have blood work results that are everywhere. This will, in general, be on the grounds that there is an awkwardness in the body, and the immune framework begins to buckle down.

It has been discovered that the main driver of numerous diseases is inflammation. Illnesses like incendiary entrail diseases, skin conditions, thyroid issues, and joint pain all follow back to the body, creating a fiery reaction in abundance.

What should be possible to normally reduce overabundance inflammation? Foods and enhancements can give a fantastic protection framework. Vegetables like tomatoes, spinach, kale, broccoli, avocados, peppers, and mushrooms ought to be consolidated into diets. Organic products like strawberries, blueberries, blackberries, raspberries, tart fruits, and oranges give valuable properties. Nuts like pecans and almonds can likewise be gainful. Healthy fats from greasy fish can give omega-3 unsaturated fats that can assist with controlling a healthy inflammation reaction, neurological procedures, and immune and cardiovascular wellbeing. Enhancements like cod liver oil from Nordic Naturals may give ideal measures of omega-3 unsaturated fats while all the while giving pivotal measures of nutrient An and D.

Proceeding onward, perceive that foods like pop, red meat, and refined starches can likewise trigger fiery reactions in the body and ought to be kept away from in huge sums.

We will, in general, consider inflammation something to be kept away from no matter what, yet recall that inflammation is a characteristic reaction actioned by our immune framework. In specific conditions, inflammation helps keep us well and shields us from contamination and tissue damage following injury.

Inflammation is normally a momentary response to something that our body deciphers as destructive, regardless of whether that is a microbe or infection, an injury from a cut or consumes or introduction to a toxin. A progression of complex compound responses happens and brings about the exemplary signs of inflammation – growing redness, heat, pain, and conceivable loss of tissue work at the injury site or injury.

In any case, when our immune framework neglects to turn off the provocative procedure, issues may happen. It is then that an acute, quick-acting response is in danger of turning into a chronic, long haul condition with a harming sway on our wellbeing and prosperity.

An anti-fiery diet can help oversee manifestations by lessening the impacts of the incendiary procedure. The diet confines certain foods while empowering others, and prescribes eating at explicit occasions to impact inflammation. Anti-incendiary diet centers around eating whole plant-based foods and fish – wealthy in healthy fats and Phyto-supplements – while balancing out glucose. In doing as such, the diet intends to impact the control instruments that deal with the incendiary procedure.

WHAT IS AN INFLAMMATORY DIET

Definition

There is nobody anti-fiery diet. Rather, there are diets structured around foods that are accepted to diminish inflammation and which avoid foods that exasperate provocative procedures. Numerous anti-inflammatory diets are based around whole grains, vegetables, nuts, seeds, crisp vegetables and organic products, wild fish and seafood, grass-took care of the fit turkey, and chicken, which are thought to help in the bodies recuperating of inflammation. They prohibit foods that are thought to trigger inflammation, for example, refined grains, wheat, corn, full-fat dairy, red meat, caffeine, liquor, peanuts, sugar, soaked, and trans-immersed fats.

The basic establishment of anti-provocative diets is the conviction that low evaluations of inflammation are the forerunner or potentially antagonizer to numerous chronic diseases. When evacuated, the body can start recuperating itself.

Starting points

The philosophical beginning of anti-provocative diets goes back to the first healers since forever who have worked with foods, herbs, teas, and other common solutions for help the body's own mending vitality.

Key terms

Chronic sickness — an ailment or ailment that keeps going over an extensive stretch of time and once in a while causes a long haul change in the body.

C-receptive protein (CRP) — a marker of inflammation flowing in the blood has been proposed as a technique to distinguish people in danger of these diseases.

Flavonoid — alludes to mixes found in organic products, vegetables, and certain refreshments that have differing useful biochemical and antioxidant impacts.

Starting during the 1970s, agents started investigating physiological systems of fever, weight misfortune, and acute stage reactions to acute and chronic contamination. Research results from these examinations started to change the standard perspectives about ailment pathogenesis. They were amassing connected proof proteins, delivered by macrophages and other immune cells, not pathogens, as once accepted, to the reason for tissue damage and infection disorders in test creatures. In this manner, the clinical calling started investigating unique treatments for chronic diseases. At that point during the 1980s, examine demonstrated that proteins, recently named cytokines, and hormone-like substances, named prostaglandins and leukotrienes, uncovered that they had pleiotropic organic exercises that were either gainful or harmful to the bodies' tissues.

From this exploration rose the cytokine hypothesis of the malady. The idea that cytokines created by the immune framework, can cause the signs, side effects, and harming delayed consequences of chronic diseases. The change didn't happen until the estimation of C-responsive protein (CRP), a marker of inflammation circling in the blood, was proposed as a strategy to recognize people in danger of chronic diseases. As spearheading research demonstrated that more elevated levels of C-responsive protein were connected to coronary illness, the ordinary idea among the clinical calling started. Initially found by W. S. Tillett and T. Francis Jr. in 1930, C-receptive protein was found as a substance in the serum of patients determined to have acute inflammation that responded with the C-polysaccharide of pneumococcus.

Today, a developing agreement among clinical experts is that inflammation is accepted to assume a job in the pathogenesis of chronic diseases, for example, coronary illness, stroke, diabetes, and colon malignant growth to give some examples. Standard reasoning is starting to acknowledge that treating the basic reason may improve cardiovascular ailment, metabolic disorder, hypertension, diabetes, and hyperlipidemia, inflammation brought about by instinctive fat tissue.

The anti-provocative diet is an eating plan intended to forestall or reduce poor quality chronic inflammation, a key hazard factor in a large group of medical issues and a few significant diseases.1

The ordinary anti-incendiary diet stresses natural products, vegetables, lean protein, nuts, seeds, and healthy fats.

General anti-fiery clinical treatments incorporate unwinding, moderate exercise, for example, strolling, weight upkeep or misfortune, and medications intended to reduce the inflammation and control the pain if present.

These medications may include ibuprofen or anti-inflammatory medicine, Non-Steroidal Anti-Inflammatory Drugs (NSAIDs), or steroid medications. The NSAIDs are broadly utilized as the underlying type of therapy. Sadly, long haul utilization of these medications can disturb the stomach and lead to ulcers. What's more, now and again can prompt kidney, just as other clinical issues.

Frequently coming about because of a way of life factors like pressure and an absence of activity, chronic inflammation results when the immune framework discharges chemicals intended to battle injury and bacterial and infection infections,2 in any event, when there are no remote intruders to fend off.

Since our food decisions impact the degree of inflammation in our bodies, the anti-provocative diet is thought to control chronic inflammation and help forestall or treat the accompanying conditions: sensitivities, Alzheimer's malady, joint pain, asthma, malignant growth, misery, diabetes, gout, coronary illness, incendiary entrail sickness, (for example, ulcerative colitis and

Crohn's ailment), bad-tempered inside disorder (IBS), and stroke. Anti-fiery diet depends on a quite solid and straightforward case: Chronic inflammation prompts chronic infection, and decreasing inflammation in the body can forestall ailment just as an advance in general wellbeing.

An anti-provocative diet expects to advance the ideal working of both cerebrum and body. It's conceivable that an anti-incendiary diet can help forestall coronary illness, numerous types of malignancy, Alzheimer's ailment, hypersensitivities, diabetes, fiery gut infection, bad-tempered inside malady (IBS), stroke, coronary illness, gout, and joint pain.

Alongside diminishing inflammation, the anti-incendiary diet is structured with the goal that individuals following the diet devour enough nutrients, minerals, fiber, essential unsaturated fats, and phytonutrients. It depends freely on the Mediterranean diet, with some deliberate increases, similar to natural tea and dim chocolate.

The anti-provocative diet isn't focused on a particular gathering of individuals. However, it very well may be especially healthy for individuals with joint pain, sensitivities, stomach related scatters, and other wellbeing intricacies that emerge from chronic inflammation.

WHAT IS INFLAMMATION

Inflammation is a restricted response of tissue to injury, regardless of whether brought about by microscopic organisms or viral disease, injury, chemicals, heat, or another marvel that causes bothering. The 'bothering' makes the tissues inside the body discharge numerous substances that cause changes inside the tissues. This unpredictable reaction is called inflammation. Inflammation is described by such manifestations that incorporate vasodilatation of the neighborhood veins bringing about overabundance nearby bloodstream, increments in the porousness of the vessels with spillage of enormous quantities of liquid into the interstitial spaces, May remember coagulating of the liquid for the interstitial spaces because of abundance measures of fibrinogen and different proteins spilling from the vessels, movement of granulocytes and monocytes into the tissue in huge quantities, in this way expanding of the tissue cells.

Inflammation has been related as a segment of, yet not restricted to, joint pain, coronary illness, diabetes, strokes, asthma, hypersensitivities, peevish entrail infection, Celiac ailment or other stomach related framework diseases, weight, chronic pressure, rest issue, for example, rest apnea, Alzheimer's malady, hypertension, raised lipids, for example, triglycerides and cholesterol.

The basic substances discharged from the tissues that bring about inflammation are histamine, bradykinin, serotonin, prostaglandins, numerous hormonal substances considered lymphokines that are discharged by sharpened T-cells, and different other response results of different frameworks inside the body. A large number of these substances actuate the macrophage framework, which is conveyed to discard the damaged tissue yet in addition, which further harms the as yet living tissue and cells.

Inflammation is an indication that the immune framework is battling the disease. The contamination might be identified with germs, wounds, allergens, toxins, or different causes.

Ordinarily, we consider signs of inflammation as redness, expanding, and pain. Be that as it may, in some cases, inflammation can occur inside our bodies. Somebody with bronchitis has a lung disease. The lungs may get aggravated. Also, this might be an indication that their immune framework is attempting to battle that disease. Excess muscle to fat ratio may advance changes in the body cells that advance chronic inflammation. The signs of inflammation may not be self-evident. For other people, chronic inflammation may identify with an issue with their immune framework.

Whatever the reason, long haul chronic inflammation may damage the body's DNA, expanding the hazard for malignant growth. Inflammation is your body's method for ensuring itself against injury and infection. Acute inflammation is significant and healthy—this is the thing that happens when you scratch your knee or sprain a lower leg. You're presumably acquainted with the redness, expanding, and warmth that joins those minor wounds.

Chronic inflammation, in any case, isn't useful for the body. Chronic inflammation can prompt a wide range of diseases, including cardiovascular infection and malignant growth, anti-provocative diet isn't generally a diet in the well-known feeling of the term. Or maybe, the anti-incendiary diet is a suggestion for a long haul eating example to accomplish and support a significant level of wellbeing.

Enrolled Dietitians, and Naturopathic doctors regularly endorse diets to diminish the fiery side effects of diseases. In spite of the fact that these diets have not been contrasted with different treatments in numerous proper research settings to date, it is felt that anti-inflammatory diets bring about a reduced measure of inflammation and a more advantageous reaction by the immune framework.

Including foods that reduce inflammation is thought to improve indications of chronic diseases and assist the decline of gambling for chronic diseases. These foods help in providing supplements that are expected to diminish inflammation. One model is omega-3 unsaturated fats. The human body utilizes these fats to fabricate prostaglandins, chemicals that assume a significant job in inflammation, and a healthy immune reaction. Another useful segment of fish oil that assumes a significant job is eicosapentaenoic corrosive (EPA), essential greasy acids.
EPA advances the creation of specific types of prostaglandins, having anti-provocative properties by lessening inflammation and diminishing the creation of fiery substances.

Intrinsic invulnerability

At the point when an individual is conceived, certain protections in the immune framework are normally present in the body. This is known as natural resistance.

It is unique in relation to versatile resistance, which we create after a disease or immunization when the body "learns" to battle a particular irresistible specialist.

Intrinsic resistance is commonly vague, while versatile insusceptibility is explicit to a specific pathogen. Inflammation is one case of an intrinsic immune reaction.

Manifestations

Manifestations of inflammation change contingent upon whether the response is acute or chronic.

The impacts of acute inflammation can be summarized by the abbreviation PARISH. They include:

- **Pain:** The exciting territory is probably going to be painful, particularly during and in the wake of contacting. Chemicals that invigorate nerve endings are discharged, making the region progressively touchy.

- **Redness:** This happens on the grounds that the vessels in the zone are loaded up with more blood than expected.

- **Immobility:** There might be some loss of capacity in the district of the inflammation.

- **Swelling:** This is brought about by the development of liquid.

- **Heat:** More bloodstreams to the influenced zone and this causes it to feel warm to the touch.

These five acute inflammation signs just apply to inflammations of the skin. On the off chance that inflammation happens somewhere inside the body, for example, in an inward organ, just a portion of the signs might be perceptible.

For instance, some inward organs might not have tactile nerve endings close by, so there will be no pain, for example, in particular types of lung inflammation.

Manifestations of chronic inflammation present in an alternate manner. These can include:

- fatigue

- mouth bruises

- chest pain

- abdominal pain

- fever

- rash

- joint pain

Causes

Inflammation is brought about by various physical responses activated by the immune framework because of a physical injury or contamination.

Inflammation doesn't really imply that there is a disease. However, contamination can cause inflammation.

Three primary procedures happen previously and during acute inflammation:

- The little parts of courses augment when providing blood to the damaged area, bringing about expanded bloodstream.

- Capillaries become simpler for liquids and proteins to penetrate, implying that they can move among blood and cells.

- The body discharges neutrophils. A neutrophil is a sort of white platelet loaded up with little sacs that contain enzymes and condensation microorganisms.

An individual will see inflammation side effects after these means occur.

Acute inflammation

Acute inflammation is one that begins quickly and gets extreme in a short space of time. Signs and indications are typically present for a couple of days yet may continue for half a month at times.

Instances of diseases, conditions, and circumstances that can bring about acute inflammation include:

- acute bronchitis

- infected ingrown toenail

- a sore throat from a cold or influenza

- a scratch or cut on the skin

- high-power work out

- acute an infected appendix

- dermatitis

- tonsillitis

- infective meningitis

- sinusitis

- a physical injury

Acute or Chronic inflammation.

Listed are the major two types of inflammation that vary in how rapidly side effects heighten and to what extent they last.

The accompanying table shows the key contrasts among acute and chronic inflammation:

Acute Chronic

Caused by Harmful microscopic organisms or tissue injury Pathogens that the body can't separate, including a few types of infection, remote bodies that stay in the framework, or overactive immune reactions

What is chronic inflammation?

This alludes to long haul inflammation and can keep going for a while and even years. It can result from:

- failure to wipe out whatever was causing an acute inflammation

- an autoimmune turmoil that attacks typical healthy tissue, confusing it with a pathogen that causes ailment

- exposure to a low degree of a specific aggravation, for example, a mechanical concoction, over a significant stretch

Instances of diseases and conditions that incorporate chronic inflammation:

- asthma

- chronic peptic ulcer

- tuberculosis

- rheumatoid joint inflammation

- periodontitis

- ulcerative colitis and Crohn's malady

- sinusitis

- active hepatitis

Albeit damaged tissue can't recuperate without inflammation, chronic inflammation can, in the long run, cause a few diseases and conditions including a few tumors, rheumatoid joint pain, atherosclerosis, periodontitis, and roughage fever.

Inflammation should be all around overseen.

Is inflammation painful?

Offer on PinterestInflammation can cause firmness and limited portability.

At the point when individuals have inflammation, it regularly stings.

Individuals will feel pain, firmness, uneasiness, trouble, and even anguish, contingent upon the seriousness of the inflammation. The sort of pain differs. It tends to be portrayed as consistent and consistent, throbbing and throbbing, cutting, or squeezing.
Inflammation essentially causes pain on the grounds that the growing pushes against the delicate nerve endings. This imparts pain signs to the mind.

Other biochemical procedures additionally happen during inflammation. They influence how nerves carry on, and this can improve pain.

Regular treatments

Inflammation is a piece of the mending procedure. Some of the time, decreasing inflammation is useful; however, not constantly essential.

Anti-provocative medications

Non-steroidal anti-provocative drugs (NSAIDs) can be taken to lighten the pain brought about by inflammation.

They check an enzyme that adds to inflammation. This either forestalls or reduces pain.

Instances of NSAIDs incorporate naproxen, ibuprofen, and anti-inflammatory medicine, which are accessible to buy on the web.

Maintain a strategic distance from the long haul utilization of NSAIDs except if exhorted by a specialist. They increment an individual's danger of stomach ulcers, which can bring about extreme, perilous dying.

NSAIDs may likewise decline asthma side effects, cause kidney damage, and increment the danger of having a stroke or coronary failure.

Acetaminophen, e.g paracetamol or Tylenol, can reduce pain without influencing the inflammation. They might be perfect for those wishing to treat only the pain while permitting the recuperating element of the inflammation to run its course.

Corticosteroids

Corticosteroids, for example, cortisol, are a class of steroid hormones that forestall various components associated with inflammation.

There are two arrangements of corticosteroids:

Glucocorticoids: These are endorsed for a scope of conditions, including:

- arthritis
- temporal arteritis
- dermatitis
- inflammatory gut illness (IBS)
- systemic lupus
- hepatitis
- asthma
- allergic responses
- sarcoidosis

Creams and treatments might be endorsed for inflammation of the skin, eyes, lungs, insides, and nose.

Mineralocorticoids: These are utilized to treat cerebral salt squandering, and to supplant significant hormones for patients with adrenal deficiency.

The symptoms of corticosteroids are almost certain whenever taken by mouth. Taking them with inhalers or infusions can reduce the hazard.

Breathed in medications, for example, those utilized long haul to treat asthma, raise the danger of creating oral thrush. Washing the mouth out with water after each utilization can help forestall oral thrush.

Glucocorticoids can likewise cause Cushing's disorder, while mineralocorticoids can cause hypertension, low blood potassium levels, connective tissue shortcoming, and issues with the degrees of acids and salts in body tissue.

Herbs for inflammation

Offer on Ginger has anti-incendiary advantages.

Talk about any conceivable utilization of homegrown enhancements with a specialist.

Harpagophytum procumbens: Also known as villain's hook, wood creepy-crawly, or catch plant, this herb originates from South Africa and is identified with sesame plants. Some exploration has indicated it might have anti-fiery properties. Different brands are accessible to buy on the web.

Hyssop: This is blended in with different herbs, for example, licorice, for the treatment of some lung conditions, including inflammation. The essential oils of hyssop can prompt hazardous spasms in research facility creatures. Alert is exhorted.

Ginger: This has been utilized for many years to treat dyspepsia, blockage, colic, and other gastrointestinal issues, just as rheumatoid joint inflammation pain. Ginger might be bought online in supplement structure.

Turmeric: Current research is investigating the conceivable useful impacts of turmeric in treating joint inflammation, Alzheimer's illness, and some other incendiary conditions. Curcumin, is a substance found in turmeric, is being contributed to the treatment of a few diseases and disarranges, including inflammation. Enhancements with turmeric and curcumin are accessible.

Cannabis: Cannabis comprises of cannabinoid called cannabichromene, which has been appeared to have

WHAT KIND OF FOOD SHOULD YOU EAT OR SHOULD NOT EAT

Anti-Inflammatory Foods to Add to Your Diet

You can help battle inflammation by eating all the more whole, nutritious foods. Characteristic foods are pressed brimming with nutrients, minerals, and fiber. These supplements help your body work all the more proficiently.

Add a greater amount of these foods to your anti-fiery diet:

- Dark, verdant greens like spinach, kale, and collards

- Fresh vegetables like broccoli, cauliflower, carrots, peppers, and tomatoes

- Healthy fats like coconut, avocados and olive oil

- Nuts like almonds, pecans, and pistachios

- Fatty fish: salmon, mackerel and fish

- Berries like strawberries, raspberries, blackberries, and blueberries

- Fresh, natural products like fruits, oranges, apples, and grapes

- Plant-based proteins like beans and lentils

- Dark chocolate

Add flavor to your meals by preparing with cinnamon, turmeric, garlic, and ginger. These herbs and flavors have amazing anti-provocative properties.

How do Anti-Inflammatory Foods Work?

Whole, characteristic foods contain a few components that can help stop or reduce inflammation. Here are some essential inflammation-battling fixings.
Crisp foods grown from the ground are pressed brimming with antioxidants. Antioxidants shield the body from free extreme damage. Free radicals are shaky molecules that cause cell damage,

malady, and inflammation. Carotenoids, found in carrots, tomatoes, and verdant green vegetables, attack inflammation. Anthocyanins, which are found in berries, keep fiery mixes from framing.

Omega-3 Fatty Acids

Cold-water fish like salmon, mackerel, and sardines are high in omega-3 unsaturated fats. These healthy fats prevent incendiary mixes from framing. They likewise reduce existing inflammation in the body.

Polyphenols

Polyphenols are a defensive plant compound. Berries, dull chocolate, herbs, and flavors are rich in polyphenols. This compound is connected to reduced inflammation in the body. Anthocyanins (a kind of polyphenol found in berries) keep incendiary mixes from framing.

Fiber

Fiber is one of the most useful supplements for powering your body. It helps lower fiery protein levels in the body. Also, fiber takes care of good microscopic organisms in the gut microbiome. This bacterial aging produces substances that reduce body-wide inflammation. Natural products, vegetables, beans, and lentils are acceptable wellsprings of fiber.

Inflammation-Causing Foods to Avoid

Certain foods and refreshments can accelerate the improvement of incendiary diseases. Also, devouring these foods and drinks can aggravate existing incendiary ailment side effects.

Cutoff your admission of the accompanying:

- Processed meats like franks, frankfurter, and bologna

- Processed snacks like chips, treats, and saltines

- Overly sweet pastries like treats, doughnuts, and dessert

- Sugary drinks like pop and squeezes

- Trans fats like shortening, vegetable oils, and seared foods

- Refined starchescarbohydrate like white bread, white rice, and white pasta

- Alcohol

FOOD THAT REDUCES CHRONIC INFLAMMATION

Whole grains

Whole grains or foods produced using them, regardless of whether split, squashed, rolled, expelled, or potentially cooked, contain the essential parts and supplements of the whole grain seed. Research has demonstrated that diets high in whole grain items are related to diminished convergences of incendiary markers and expanded adiponectin levels. The defensive impacts of a diet high in whole grains on fundamental inflammation might be clarified, to a limited extent, by the decrease in overproduction of oxidative pressure that outcomes in inflammation.

Whole grain will incorporate the accompanying pieces of the grain bit—the wheat, germ, and endosperm. Such whole grains are amaranth, grain, bulgur, wild rice, millet, oats, quinoa, rye, spelled, wheat berries, buckwheat, and whole wheat.

Vegetables

Diets high in vegetables are conversely identified with plasma centralizations of C-receptive protein (CRP). Among the numerous assortments of vegetables are; pinto beans, lentils, kidney beans, borlotti beans, mung beans, soybeans, cannelloni beans, garbanzo or chickpeas, adzuki beans, fava beans, and dark beans.

Nuts, seeds

Nuts and seeds are wealthy in unsaturated fat and different supplements that may reduce inflammation. Visit nut utilization is related to lower levels of provocative markers. This may clarify why there is a lower danger of cardiovascular infection and type 2 diabetes with visit nut and seed utilization. Except for peanuts, make certain to include pecans, flax seeds, and pumpkin seeds. The Nuts and seeds are best eaten when unsalted and crude.

New vegetables

Green verdant vegetables and brilliantly shaded vegetables give beta-carotene; nutrient C and different antioxidants have been appeared to reduce cell damage and to have anti-incendiary impacts. Focus on at least three servings every day.

New natural products

Flavonoids found in new natural products among different substances are thought to build the antioxidant impacts of nutrient C. look into has indicated that organic products have an anti-incendiary impact. Focus on at least two servings every day. Make certain to remember berries for your week after week selections of organic products, for example, blueberries, blackberries, and strawberries.

Wild fish and seafood

Slick fish, for example, Herring, Mackerel, Salmon, and Trout are a phenomenal wellspring of omega-3 unsaturated fats, as are shellfish, for example, mussels and mollusks. Remembering fish or seafood high for omega-3 unsaturated fats at any rate three times each week is suggested.

Lean poultry

Protein is utilized in the body to fix and production cells, make antibodies, enzymes, and hormones. Lean protein has been related to lower levels of fiery biomarkers.

While picking poultry, pick grass-took care of creatures, which will, in general, have a higher measure of essential unsaturated fats—select poultry with restricted measures of, or liberated from, additives, sodium, nitrates or shading. Additionally, in a perfect diet, just 10-12 percent of everyday calories should originate from protein. All things considered, a grown-up needs 0.36 grams of protein per pound of body weight.

Soy items

Anti-incendiary properties of the isoflavones, a micronutrient segment of soy, have been accounted for in a few exploratory models and sickness conditions.

The information recommends the chance of valuable impacts of isoflavone-rich soy foods when added to the diet. Soy items incorporate; soybeans, edema me, tofu, tempeh, soymilk, just as numerous different items produced using soybeans.

Oils

Expeller squeezed Canola oil, and Extra Virgin Olive oil is types of oil that have been connected to reduced inflammation. Different oils thought to help in diminishing inflammation incorporate rice-wheat, grape seed, evening primrose, and pecan oil. It is proposed to utilize these oils with some restraint when cooking, heating, and enhancing of foods. Additionally, when buying oils, ensure they are unadulterated oils as opposed to mixed oils. Mixed oil, for the most part, contains less stimulating oils.

Water as crisp drinking water liberated from harmful chemicals.

Water is an essential substance for each capacity of the body. It is a mode for substance forms; a dissolvable for body squander and weakens their lethality and helps in their discharge. Water helps in ingestion, retention, and transport of indispensable supplements that have anti-fiery impacts. Water is additionally required for fundamental cell working, fixing of body tissues, and is the base of all blood and liquid discharges.

Herbs and Spices

A greater measure of research is rising on the antioxidant properties of herbs and flavors and their utilization in the administration of chronic inflammation. Herbs and flavors can be utilized in recipes to halfway or entirely supplant less attractive fixings, for example, salt, sugar and included immersed fat, know for their incendiary impacts, in this manner decreasing the harming properties of these foods.

Safeguards

Foods that disturb inflammation

Best alluded to in look into books as 'the western dietary example,' it credits a diet that is high in refined grains, red meat, margarine, handled meats, high-fat dairy, desserts and sweets, pizza, potato, eggs, hydrogenated fats, and soda pops. This example of eating is emphatically identified with an expansion in coursing blood CRP levels and greater dangers for chronic diseases, weight, and tumors. These foods, named 'professional incendiary,' may expand inflammation, in this way, expanding a people hazard for chronic diseases just as fuel manifestations from these chronic conditions.

There is some help for the conviction that food sensitivities or allergens to foods might be a trigger for inflammation. Regularly difficult to identify with normal blood tests, a few people have seen lightening of indications of chronic diseases, for example, joint pain, when the irritating foods are expelled from their diet. Regular unfavorably susceptible foods are milk and dairy, wheat, corn, eggs, meat, yeast, and soy.

Other stars incendiary foods have been appeared to have substances that actuate or bolster the fiery procedure. Unhealthy trans fats and immersed fats utilized in getting ready and handling certain foods are connected to expanded inflammation. Handled meats, for example, lunchmeats, wieners, and hotdogs, contain chemicals, for example, nitrites that are related to expanded inflammation and chronic malady.

Soaked fats normally found in meats, dairy items, and eggs contain unsaturated fats called arachidonic corrosive. While some arachidonic corrosive is essential for wellbeing, abundance arachidonic corrosive in the diet has been appeared to intensify inflammation.

Research bolsters that diets high in sugar produce acute oxidative worry inside the cells, partner it with inflammation. End of high sugar foods, for example, soft drinks, soda pops, cakes, presweetened grains, and candy has been demonstrated to be gainful. Just as changing from refined grains to whole grains.

A Food List of What to Eat and Avoid on an Anti-Inflammatory Diet

Following an anti-fiery diet implies stacking up on foods that exploration has indicated can help lower inflammation, and lessening your admission of foods that have the contrary impact. Probably the best thing about the diet is there are a lot of food alternatives and bunches of squirm room, so you can single out the foods you like best.

In the event that you need somewhat more structure, consider embracing the Mediterranean diet. There's a great deal of cover with the anti-incendiary diet in light of the fact that both underline eating natural products, vegetables, and whole grains.

Foods to Eat

- Fresh, natural product, including grapefruit, grapes, blueberries, bananas, apples, mangoes, peaches, tomatoes, and pomegranates

- Dried natural product, including plums

- Vegetables, particularly broccoli, Brussels sprouts, cauliflower, and bok choy

- Plant-based proteins, for example, chickpeas, seitan, and lentils.

- Fatty fish, for example, salmon, sardines, tuna fish, herring, lake trout, and mackerel.

- Whole grains, including oatmeal, dark colored rice, grain, and whole-wheat bread

- Leafy greens, including kale, spinach, and romaine lettuce

- Ginger

- Nuts, including pecans and almonds

- Seeds, for example, chia seeds and flaxseed.

- Foods loaded up with omega-3 unsaturated fats, for example, avocado and olive oil.

- Coffee

- Green tea

- Dark chocolate (with some restraint)

- Red wine (with some restraint)

Foods to Eat Sparingly or Avoid

- Refined sugars, for example, white bread, baked goods, and desserts.

- The Foods and beverages which are high in sugar, including pop and other sugary refreshments

- Red meat

- Dairy

- Processed meat, for example, franks and frankfurters.

- Fried foods

12 THINGS YOU NEED TO KNOW ABOUT ANTI-INFLAMMATORY DIETS

Anti-fiery foods are getting huge amounts of promotion nowadays. Truth be told, pretty much everybody is utilizing the expression "inflammation," from your cardiologist to Tom and Gisele! Be that as it may, keep your baloney indicator on. This is the thing that anti-fiery diets really are — and aren't — about.

1. Inflammatory diets are additionally a thing.

The soaked fat included sugar and sodium in refined carbs, and handled tidbits make your body's cells stay at work longer than required to complete their standard occupation. Specialists can distinguish inflammation utilizing biomarkers of oxidative pressure, the consequence of natural procedures that cause organ tissue damage. Diet, exercise, and smoking status can influence inflammation, however, so do wild causes like autoimmune diseases.

2. It's not only for weight misfortune.

Anti-provocative eating is, to a greater extent, a malady counteraction plan. A mind-boggling measure of research has demonstrated that individuals who eat anti-provocative foods are at essentially lower danger of creating chronic malady. They're additionally bound to keep up healthy weights.

3. Anti-incendiary foods are all over the place.

The anti-incendiary diet is frequently viewed as a Mediterranean diet since they suggest comparative foods: Veggies, natural products, whole grains, nuts, seeds, oils, vegetables, low-fat dairy, and fish. The flavonoids in plants are explicitly connected to shielding your body's cells from damage. Both produce and lean protein sources like beans and seafood likewise contain bravo polyunsaturated and monounsaturated fats.

4. You may have these shrouded signs of inflammation.

You can't feel inflammation in any case, in the event that you recognize what manifestations to search for, you can get it right on time before wellbeing conditions develop. As indicated by – creator of the Whole Body Cure, a leap forward program shows you how to reduce inflammation. Potential provocative admonition signs incorporate stomach related problems, discontinuous joint pain, new food sensitivities, gut fat, exacerbating hypersensitivities, cerebrum mist, unexplained weakness, grumpiness, rest issues, and rashes.

5. It's comprehensive, not elite.

Conventional diets consistently talk about what you can't eat, yet with regards to anti-fiery diets, more will be more. Bright foods like verdant greens (spinach, kale), cruciferous veggies (broccoli, cauliflower), carotenoids (tomatoes, carrots), and anthocyanins (beets, berries) are on the whole anti-fiery staples.

6. You won't feel hungry.

The plant-based powerhouses known as heartbeats are an amazing method to fuse antioxidant-and mineral-rich foods into your regular daily existence. Dry peas, beans, chickpeas, and lentils consolidate lean protein, unsaturated fats, and fiber, topping you off without upsetting your diet.

7. Wine and espresso are energized.

With regards to diminishing your danger of Alzheimer's, cardiovascular ailment and diabetes, light to direct liquor admission of any sort can help. Pressed with flavonoids and antioxidants, espresso beans avert subjective decay, yet additionally, support cerebrum capacity and incitement of the focal sensory system. Simply avoid improved beverages — sugary refreshments can expand inflammation!

8. Your state of mind could get a lift.

Ladies of childbearing age eat half less fish than they should, to a great extent because of past perplexity about pre-birth impacts. Actually, 12 ounces of seven days can give a whole host of anti-incendiary advantages. In addition, the omega-3's in fish have been connected to a lower danger of misery and reduced nervousness indications. A portion of our preferred picks incorporates fish, salmon, sardines, anchovies, and other white fish.

9. it's loaded up with enhance.

Turmeric offers incredible anti provocative advantages, of the Whole Body Cure, an anti-fiery diet plan from our accomplices at Prevention. Supercharge its anti-incendiary impacts by joining it with dark pepper, which assists with expanding the measure of curcumin (the dynamic fixing in turmeric) your body can assimilate. Turmeric is additionally fat solvent, he says, so you'll expand your assimilation by consolidating it with a healthy fat like olive oil.

10. Cooking oils are OK.

Extra-virgin olive oil is loaded up with polyphenols, antioxidant-mixes connected to keeping up cell uprightness and improving bloodstream all through your body. Canola oil, produced using rapeseed, is another anti-incendiary staple.

11. Conscious guilty pleasures are critical.

At last, the anti-provocative diet stresses genuine foods as close to nature as could be expected under the circumstances. Be that as it may, since extravagance is a key piece of any eating plan, take a stab at treating yourself to around 200 calories of chocolate for every day. Research says that eating chocolate consistently may likewise help keep up an ordinary BMI. Additionally, it can assist you with curtailing other handled treats.

12. You can attempt a whole-body approach.

Counteraction's Whole Body Cure incorporates 60+ anti-incendiary recipes. Alongside the nitty-gritty counsel, you have to invert chronic inflammation — no solution required.

WHAT KIND OF DISEASE CAN INFLAMMATION CAUSE

Instances of diseases and conditions that incorporate chronic inflammation:

- Asthma.

- Chronic peptic ulcer.

- Tuberculosis.

- Rheumatoid joint inflammation.

- Periodontitis.

- Ulcerative colitis and Crohn's ailment.

- Sinusitis.

- Active hepatitis.

1. ASTHMA

WHAT IS MEANT BY "INFLAMMATION" IN ASTHMA?

To an ever-increasing extent, we hear talk about "inflammation" in asthma. Our perspective on what asthma is has changed over the previous decade or thereabouts. Never again is the emphasis solely on narrowing of the breathing ways (bronchial cylinders) because of constriction of the bronchial muscles that encompass these cylinders. Progressively, there is an accentuation on the significance of inflammation of the bronchial cylinders and treatment with medications that reduce this inflammation (anti-fiery drugs). This handout examines what is implied by inflammation in asthma, and why it is so imperative to treat inflammation in asthma, regardless of whether it isn't causing us any indications, for example, hack or wheeze or brevity of breath.

Different Examples of Inflammation

Inflammation is a term utilized in medication to portray how the body responds to different types of injury or aggravation or contamination. Inflammation takes different structures. A burn from the sun is a kind of inflammation of the skin in response to the bright beams of daylight. The rash of toxic substance ivy is another sort of inflammation of the skin, an unfavorably susceptible response to oils on the leaves of the toxic substance ivy plant.

Inflammation Can be Acute or Chronic

Like these two models, a few types of inflammation keep going for just a brief while and afterward leave when the reason for the aggravation is evacuated. In any case, different types of inflammation can keep going for quite a long time or years or even a lifetime. As yet thinking about inflammation of the skin, psoriasis is a case of dependable or chronic inflammation. Rheumatoid joint inflammation is a chronic provocative illness of the joints of the body.

Regardless of whether it is brief (acute) or dependable (chronic), inflammation can leave suddenly and completely. Different occasions, inflammation can abandon scarring and perpetual changes in the body system.

Asthma Attacks And The Bronchial Tubes Acute Inflammation

It's known for quite a while that acute inflammation of the bronchial cylinders happens during asthma attacks. The bronchial cylinders become swollen and limited, and bodily fluid is discharged into the cylinders from organs in the dividers of the cylinders. Growing of the cylinders and their stopping with bodily fluid make it hard to breathe. You may hack up a portion of this thick, gooey bodily fluid during a flare of your asthma.

Asthma is a Chronic Inflammation condition of the Bronchial Tubes

A significant clinical disclosure quite a while prior was that some inflammation is available in the bronchial containers of people with asthma in any event, when they feel well and when their breathing is typical. The reason for this chronic inflammation isn't known, despite the fact that on numerous occasions, it resembles an unfavorably susceptible kind of response. The inflammation might be gentle, so mellow that it doesn't cause narrowing of the bronchial cylinders. In any case, the persevering or chronic nearness of the inflammation most likely is the thing that makes the bronchial cylinders fit for narrowing strangely. The bronchial cylinders in asthma are said to be "jittery" or effortlessly sent into fit or narrowing. What makes the bronchial cylinders "jumpy" or helpless against an assortment of boosts in our general surroundings, whether it be residue or exercise or feline dander or cold air-is believed to be the relentless nearness of inflammation in the bronchial cylinders.

Approaches to Reduce Inflammation in Asthma

There are, notwithstanding, two head approaches to reduce it. The first is to distinguish those things that are invigorating the inflammation in any case and freeing them from the earth, which means by and large from the air that we breathe. A few things, similar to tobacco smoke and air contamination, are probably going to exacerbate the inflammation of the bronchial cylinders in anybody with asthma. Different things, similar to feline dander or house dust, cause asthmatic inflammation just in those people who are explicitly sensitive to felines or residue. Here and there, sensitivity testing is utilized to recognize those things to which an individual is unfavorably susceptible with the objective of lessening or taking out the measure of presentation to them.

Medications That Can Reduce the Inflammation of the Bronchial Tubes

The other head approach to reduce the chronic inflammation of the bronchial cylinders is to take medications that smother it. These are the anti-fiery medications of asthma. For long haul use, at present three unique types of anti-provocative medications are accessible to treat asthma: cromolyn (brand name: Intal®), nedocromil (brand name: Tilade®), and the breathed in corticosteroids (brand names: Aerobid®, Flovent®, Pulmicort®, Qvar®,Azmacort®, Beclovent®, and Vanceril®). These listed medications can keep the inflammation of the bronchial cylinders at any rate while you take them; on the off chance that you stop the anti-provocative medications, the inflammation of the bronchial cylinders, as a rule, returns inside half a month to what it was before taking the medications.

The "Non-Steroidal Anti-Inflammatory Medications" Do Not Work for Asthmatic Inflammation

One kind of anti-provocative medication works for the inflammation of joint pain; however, it isn't powerful in asthma. These are known as the "non-steroidal anti-fiery drugs" or NSAIDs. Models incorporate headache medicine, ibuprofen, naproxen, Motrin®, Naprosyn®, Ansaid®, Tolectin®, and numerous others. In addition to the fact that these groups of medications did not assist with treating the inflammation of asthma, in certain people with asthma—those with an affectability to ibuprofen—these meds can welcome on an attack of asthma, frequently one that is very extreme.

Preventive Treatment in Asthma

When growing of the bronchial cylinders and extreme bodily fluid creation cause hack and wheezing and brevity of breath, the anti-fiery medications can reduce these side effects by lessening inflammation in the bronchial cylinders. In any case, for what reason is it suggested for some people with asthma that they take their anti-provocative medications consistently, in any event, when feeling admirable? By decreasing the inflammation that is available, the "jumpiness" of the bronchial cylinders diminishes. One turns out to be less powerless against the chance of building up an attack of asthma from the growing and fit of the bronchial cylinders. Anti-incendiary medications are defensive or preventive. They are utilized each day to keep the side effects of asthma from creating. The objective of effective asthma care is to keep the manifestations of asthma from growing instead of alleviating them with medications once they happen.

The Anti-Inflammatory Medications Are Safe to Use Every Day

The medications used to treat inflammation in asthma have been being used for over 30 years. They are accepted to be sheltered when utilized each day: they don't lose their viability after some time, they don't make you become subordinate ("dependent") to them, and they don't mess clinical up much following quite a while of utilization.

2. CHRONIC PEPTIC ULCER

• A peptic ulcer is bruised in the covering of the throat, stomach, or duodenum.

• The principal indication of a stomach or duodenal ulcer is upper stomach pain, which can be dull, sharp, or consuming (a yearning like inclination). (Swelling and burping are not side effects of peptic ulcer, and heaving, poor craving, and queasiness are remarkable indications of peptic ulcer.)

• Other related side effects may include:

o Acid reflux or indigestion

o Feeling satisfied (full) when eating

• Peptic ulcer arrangement is identified with H. pylori microscopic organisms in the stomach and nonsteroidal anti-fiery medications (NSAIDs) in half of the patients. For the staying half, there are incidental causes, for example, drugs, way of life factors (smoking), extreme physiological pressure, and hereditary elements, yet less as often as possible, the reason is obscure.

• Ulcer pain may not connect with the nearness or seriousness of ulceration.

• The Diagnosis of an ulcer can be made with an upper GI arrangement or endoscopy.

• Treatment of the throat, stomach, or duodenal ulcersaims to diminish pain, mend the ulcer, and forestall confusion. Clinical treatment includes antibiotic blends alongside stomach corrosive concealment medication, for instance, acid neutralizers, proton siphon inhibitors (PPIs) to annihilate H. pylori disposing of accelerating elements, for example, NSAIDs or smothering stomach corrosive alone.

• Complications of esophageal, duodenal or stomach ulcers incorporate;

o bleeding,

o perforation, and

o blockage to the entry of food because of a gastric check from the expanding or frightening that encompasses the ulcer.

• If an individual with peptic ulcers smokes or takes NSAIDs, the ulcers may repeat after treatment.

Draining Ulcers Symptoms and Causes

Draining ulcers are a serious deal. Frequently having endoscopy is demonstrative and helpful. A gastroenterologist can utilize a fiberoptic camera to see within the stomach and duodenum, scanning for a wellspring of dying.

Manifestations of a draining ulcer include:

• Indigestion

• Abdominal distress in the wake of eating

• Upper stomach consuming or hunger pain 1 to 3 hours subsequent to eating or in the night

What a peptic ulcer is?

The peptic ulcer (stomach or duodenal) is a break in the inward covering of the throat, stomach, or duodenum. A peptic ulcer of the stomach is known as a gastric ulcer; of the duodenum, a duodenal ulcer; and of the throat and esophageal ulcer. Peptic ulcers happen when the coating these organs is dissolved by the acidic stomach related (peptic) juices that the cells of the covering discharge of the stomach emit. A peptic ulcer varies from a disintegration since it expands further into the covering and impels a greater amount of an incendiary response from the tissues that are included, every so often with startling. Peptic ulcer additionally is alluded to as peptic ulcer sickness.

Peptic ulcer infection is normal, influencing a great many Americans yearly. Additionally, peptic ulcers are a repetitive issue; even mended ulcers can repeat except if treatment is aimed at forestalling their repeat. The clinical expense of treating peptic ulcers and its intricacies runs into billions of dollars every year. Ongoing clinical advances have expanded our comprehension of ulcer development. Improved and extended treatment choices presently are accessible.

Are peptic ulcers painful?

The pain of ulcer ailment relates ineffectively with the nearness or seriousness of dynamic ulceration. A few people have tenacious pain considerably after an ulcer is totally mended by medication. Others experience no pain by any means. Ulcers frequently travel every which way precipitously without the individual ever realizing that they are available except if a genuine difficulty (like draining or puncturing) happens.

What are the early signs and side effects of peptic ulcers?

Side effects and signs of peptic (esophageal, duodenal, or stomach) ulcers malady fluctuate. A few people with stomach ulcers don't have any manifestations or signs, while others may have a couple or a few.

The most widely recognized manifestation of a peptic ulcer is a dull or consuming pain in the stomach. The pain might be felt anyplace between your gut catch and breastbone. Pain from a peptic or stomach ulcer;

1. Usually happens when your stomach is unfilled, for instance, for example, between meals or during the night;

2. May stop quickly in the event that you eat or take stomach settling agents;

3. May keep going for a considerable length of time to hours;

4. May go back and forth for a few days, weeks, or months

Peptic ulcer different side effects and signs that are less regular incorporate;
  a. bloating,

  b. burping,

  c. feeling debilitated to your stomach,

  d. poor hunger,

  e. vomiting, and

  f. weight misfortune.

Regardless of whether your manifestations are gentle, you may have a peptic ulcer. You should see your primary care physician discuss your manifestations. Without treatment, your peptic ulcer can deteriorate.

What causes peptic ulcers?

For a long time, overabundance corrosive was accepted to be a significant reason for ulcer ailment. As needs are, the accentuation of treatment was on killing and repressing the emission of stomach corrosive. While corrosive is as yet viewed as essential for the development of ulcers and its concealment is as yet the essential treatment, the two most significant starting reasons for ulcers is disease of the stomach by a bacterium named "Helicobacter pylori" (H. pylori) and chronic utilization of nonsteroidal anti-provocative medications or NSAIDs, including headache medicine. Cigarette smoking additionally is a significant reason for ulcers just as a disappointment of ulcer mending.

Disease with H. pylori is normal, influencing in excess of a billion people around the world. It is evaluated that half of the United States populace more seasoned than age 60 has been contaminated with H. pylori. Contamination typically endures for a long time, prompting ulcer malady in 10% to 15% of those tainted. Before, H. pylori were found in over 80% of patients with gastric and duodenal ulcers. With expanding gratefulness, diagnosis, and treatment of this contamination, the predominance of disease with H. pylori just as the extent of ulcers brought about by the bacterium has diminished. It is evaluated that right now, just 20% of ulcers are related to the bacterium. While the component by which H. pylori causes ulcers is perplexing, end of the bacterium by antibiotics has obviously been appeared to mend ulcers and forestall their repeat.

NSAIDs are medications utilized for the treatment of joint pain and other painful provocative conditions in the body. Headache medicine, ibuprofen (Advil, Motrin), naproxen (Aleve, Naprosyn), and etodolac (Lodine) are a couple of instances of this class of medications. Prostaglandins are substances delivered by the body, which are significant in helping the linings of the throat, stomach, and duodenum to oppose damage by the acidic stomach related juices of the stomach. NSAIDs cause ulcers by meddling with the creation of prostaglandins in the stomach.

Cigarette smoking causes ulcers. However, it additionally builds the danger of intricacies from ulcers, for example, dying, obstacle, and puncturing. Cigarette smoking additionally is the main source of the disappointment of treatment for ulcers.

As opposed to prevalent thinking, liquor, espresso, colas, hot foods, and caffeine have no demonstrated job in ulcer arrangement. Additionally, there is no indisputable proof to recommend that life stresses or character types add to ulcer illness.

Methods and tests to analyze peptic ulcers.

The diagnosis of an ulcer is carried out by either a barium upper gastrointestinal X-beam (upper GI arrangement) or an upper gastrointestinal endoscopy (EGD or esophagogastroduodenoscopy). The barium upper gastrointestinal (GI) X-beam is anything but difficult to perform and includes no hazard (other than an introduction to radiation) or inconvenience. Barium is a white substance that is gulped. It is noticeable on X-beams and permits the framework of the stomach to be seen on X-beams; in any case, barium X-beams are less exact and may miss ulcers up to 20% of the time.

An upper gastrointestinal endoscopy is more exact than X-beams, yet as a rule includes sedation of the patient and the inclusion of an adaptable cylinder through the mouth to examine the throat, stomach, and duodenum. Upper endoscopy has the additional bit of leeway of having the ability to evacuate little tissue tests (biopsies) to test for H. pylori disease. Biopsies are likewise inspected under a magnifying instrument to prohibit a destructive ulcer. While for all intents and purposes, every single duodenal ulcer is kind, gastric ulcers can, at times, be destructive. In this way, biopsies frequently are performed on gastric ulcers to avoid malignancy.

Is there a diet for peptic ulcers? Would you be able to drink liquor?

There is no decisive proof that dietary limitations and tasteless diets assume a job in ulcer was recuperating. No demonstrated relationship exists between peptic ulcer ailment and the admission of espresso and liquor. In any case, since espresso animates corrosive gastric discharge, and liquor can cause gastritis, balance in liquor and espresso utilization is suggested.

What is the treatment for peptic ulcers?

The objective of ulcer treatment is to assuage pain, recuperate the ulcer, and forestall confusion. The initial phase in treatment includes a decrease in hazard factors (NSAIDs and cigarettes). The following stage is medications.

H. pylori treatment

Numerous individuals harbor H. pylori in their stomachs while never having pain or ulcers. It isn't totally certain whether these patients ought to be treated with antibiotics. More examinations are expected to address this inquiry.

• Patients with reported ulcer ailment and H. pylori contamination ought to be treated for both the ulcer and the H. pylori. H. pylori can be extremely hard to totally destroy.

• Treatment for peptic ulcers requires a blend of a few antibiotics, in some cases in a mix with a proton-siphon inhibitor, H2 blockers, or Pepto-Bismol.

• Commonly utilized antibiotics are;

  • tetracycline,

  • amoxicillin,

  • metronidazole (Flagyl),

  • clarithromycin (Biaxin), and

  • levofloxacin (Levaquin).

Annihilation of H. pylori forestalls the arrival of ulcers (a significant issue with all other ulcer treatment alternatives). Disposal of these microorganisms additionally may diminish the danger of creating gastric malignant growth later on.

Treatment with antibiotics conveys the danger of unfavorably susceptible responses, looseness of the bowels, and now and again extreme antibiotic-prompted colitis (inflammation of the colon). What are the confusions of peptic ulcers?

With current treatment, individuals with ulcer infection can have ordinary existences without the way of life changes or dietary limitations. Cigarette and cannabis smokers have been found to have more complexities from ulcers and treatment failures.

Destruction of the microscopic organisms H. pylori recuperates ulcers as well as forestalls the repeat of ulcer sickness.

Patients with ulcers, for the most part, work easily.

A few ulcers likely recuperate even without medications (however, they presumably repeat also). Along these lines, the serious issues coming about because of ulcers are identified with ulcer complexities. Entanglements incorporate;

• bleeding,

• perforation, and

• Obstruction of purging of the entry of food.

Patients with draining ulcers may report;

• passage of dark delay stools (melena),

• weakness,

• a feeling of wooziness or ay even drop after standing (orthostatic hypotension or syncope),

• and spewing blood (hematemesis). Starting treatment includes the quick substitution of liquids intravenously.

Patients with industrious or extreme draining may require blood transfusions. An endoscopy is performed to build up the site of draining and to stop dynamic ulcer seeping with the guide of particular endoscopic instruments.

An aperture through the stomach prompts the spillage of stomach substance into the stomach (peritoneal) pit, bringing about acute peritonitis (disease of the stomach cavity). These patients report an abrupt beginning of outrageous stomach pain, which is compounded by a movement. Stomach muscles become inflexible and board-like. Earnest medical procedures normally are required. A duodenal ulcer that has punctured can tunnel into neighboring organs, for example, the pancreas or behind the guts and into the back. An esophageal ulcer that punctures can cause extreme inflammation of the tissues that encompass it (mediastinitis).

Duodenum - A peptic ulcer that structures in the thin outlet from the stomach, it can impede the progression of stomach substance into the duodenum. Duodenal ulcers, in some cases, additionally may impede the progression of intestinal substance.

Patients with check frequently report;

• increasing stomach pain,

• vomiting of undigested or halfway processed food,

• diminished craving, and

• Weight misfortune.

The check fo,r the most part ha, opens at or approach the pylorus of the stomach. Endoscopy is helpful in building up the diagnosis of hindrance from cancer and barring gastric cancer as a reason for the check. In certain patients, gastric deterrent can be assuaged by such notion of the stomach substance with a cylinder for 72 hours, alongside intravenous anti-ulcer medications, for example, cimetidine (Tagamet) and ranitidine (Zantac).

What is the forecast for an individual with peptic ulcer sickness? Would it be able to be restored?

With current treatment, individuals with ulcer ailment can have typical existences without the way of life changes or dietary limitations. Cigarette smokers have been found to have more inconveniences from ulcers and treatment disappointment. Destruction of the microscopic organisms H. pylori mends ulcers as well as forestalls the repeat of ulcer illness.

Which fortes of specialists treat peptic ulcers?

Specialists who normally treat peptic ulcer infection incorporate essential consideration suppliers, for example, general medication doctors, family medication specialists, and internists. Experts in the diagnosis and treatment of peptic ulcer ailment are gastroenterologists.

3. TUBERCULOSIS

Tuberculosis (TB) is an irresistible ailment that normally influences the lungs. However, it can influence any organ in the body. It can create when microbes spread through beads noticeable all around. TB can be deadly; however, by and large, it is preventable and treatable.

What is tuberculosis?

An individual with TB may encounter swollen lymph hubs.

An individual may create TB in the wake of breathing in Mycobacterium tuberculosis (M. tuberculosis) microbes.

At the point when TB influences the lungs, the malady is the most infectious. However, an individual will generally just get debilitated after close contact with somebody who has this sort of TB.

TB disease (idle TB)

An individual can have TB microorganisms in their body and never create indications. In a great many people, the immune framework can contain the microbes with the goal that they don't reproduce and cause infection. Right now, the individual will have TB contamination, yet not the dynamic infection.

Specialists allude to this as inert TB. An individual may never encounter indications and be uninformed that they have the disease. There is likewise no danger of giving dormant contamination to someone else. In any case, an individual with inert TB despite everything requires treatment.

The CDC gauge that upwards of 13 million individuals in the U.S. have dormant TB.

TB illness (dynamic TB)

The body might not be able to contain TB microorganisms. This is progressively normal when the immune framework is debilitated because of sickness or the utilization of specific medications.

At the point when this occurs, the microscopic organisms can recreate and cause manifestations, bringing about dynamic TB. Individuals with dynamic TB can spread contamination.

Without clinical intercession, TB gets dynamic in 5–10% of individuals with the disease. In about half of these individuals, the movement happens inside 2–5 years of getting the contamination, as indicated by the CDC.

The danger of creating dynamic TB is greater in:

- anyone with a debilitated immune framework

- anyone who originally built up the disease in the previous 2–5 years

- older grown-ups and little youngsters

- people who utilize infused recreational drugs

- people who have not gotten suitable treatment for TB before

Early admonition signs

An individual should see a specialist on the off chance that they experience:

- a diligent hack, enduring at any rate 3 weeks

- phlegm, which may have blood in it, when they hack

- a loss of hunger and weight

- a general sentiment of weariness and being unwell

- swelling in the neck

- a fever

- night sweats

- chest pain

Manifestations

Inert TB: An individual with idle TB will have no side effects, and no damage will appear on a chest X-beam. Nonetheless, a blood test or skin prick test will demonstrate that they have TB contamination.

Dynamic TB: An individual with TB malady may encounter a hack that produces mucus, weakness, a fever, chills, and lost craving and weight. Indications ordinarily exacerbate after some time. However, they can likewise suddenly leave and return.

Past the lungs

TB generally influences the lungs. However, side effects can create different pieces of the body. This is increasingly basic in individuals with debilitated immune frameworks.

TB can cause:

- persistently swollen lymph hubs, or "swollen organs."

- abdominal pain

- joint or bone pain

- confusion

- an industrious migraine

- seizures

Diagnosis

An individual with dormant TB will have no indications, yet the disease can appear on tests. Individuals ought to request a TB test on the off chance that they:

- have invested energy with an individual who has or is in danger of TB

- have invested energy in a nation with high paces of TB

- work in a situation where TB might be available

A specialist will get some information about any indications and the individual's clinical history. They will likewise play out a physical assessment, which includes tuning in to the lungs and checking for expanding in the lymph hubs.

Two tests can show whether TB microscopic organisms are available:

- the TB skin test

- the TB blood test

Be that as it may, these can't demonstrate whether TB is dynamic or inert. To test for dynamic TB illness, the specialist may prescribe a sputum test and a chest X-beam.

Everybody with TB needs treatment, whether or not the contamination is dynamic or inert.

Treatment

With early recognition and proper antibiotics, TB is treatable.

The correct sort of antibiotic and length of treatment will rely upon:

- the individual's age and general wellbeing

- whether they have idle or dynamic TB

- the area of the disease

- whether the strain of TB is drug safe

Treatment for idle TB can fluctuate. It might include taking an antibiotic once per week for 12 weeks or consistently for 9 months.

Treatment for dynamic TB may include consuming a few medications for 6–9 months. At the point when an individual has a drug safe strain of TB, the treatment will be increasingly intricate.

It is essential to finish the full course of treatment, regardless of whether manifestations leave. In the event that an individual quits taking their medication early, a few microscopic organisms can endure and get impervious to antibiotics. Right now, the individual may proceed to create safe drug TB.

Contingent upon the pieces of the body that TB influences, a specialist may likewise recommend corticosteroids.

Causes

M. tuberculosis microscopic organisms cause TB. They can spread through the air in beads when an individual with pneumonic TB hacks, sniffles, spits, giggles, or talks.

Just individuals with dynamic TB can transmit the disease. Many people with the illness can never again transmit the microscopic organisms after they have gotten suitable treatment for at any rate 2 weeks.

Counteraction

Methods for keeping TB from tainting others include:

• getting a diagnosis and treatment early

• staying endlessly from others until there is never again a danger of disease

• wearing a veil, covering the mouth, and ventilating rooms

4. RHEUMATOID ARTHRITIS

Specialists call an autoimmune condition. It begins when your immune framework, which should secure you, goes astray, and starts to attack your body's own tissues. It causes inflammation in the coating of your joints (the synovium). Subsequently, your joints may get red, warm, swollen, and painful.

RA influences joints on the two sides of the body, for example, two hands, the two wrists, or the two knees. This evenness assists with separating it from different types of joint pain. After some time, RA can influence other body parts and frameworks, from your eyes to your heart, lungs, skin, veins, and that's only the tip of the iceberg.

Manifestations of Rheumatoid Arthritis

The admonition signs of RA are:

• Joint pain and growing

• Stiffness of the body, particularly toward the beginning of the day or after you sit for quite a while

• Fatigue

Rheumatoid joint inflammation influences everybody in an unexpected way. For a few, joint side effects happen progressively more than quite a while. In others, it might come on rapidly.

A few people may have rheumatoid joint inflammation for a brief timeframe and afterward go into abatement, which implies they don't have indications.

Who Gets Rheumatoid Arthritis?

Anybody can get RA. It influences about 1% of Americans.

The illness is 2 to multiple times more typical in ladies than in men, yet men will, in general, have progressively serious indications.

It, as a rule, begins in middle age. Be that as it may, little youngsters and the older additionally can get it.

Reasons for Rheumatoid Arthritis

Specialists don't have the foggiest idea about the specific reason. Something appears to trigger the immune framework to attack your joints and, now and then, different organs. A few specialists figure an infection or microbes may change your immune framework, making it attack your joints. Different speculations recommend that in certain individuals, smoking may prompt rheumatoid joint inflammation.

Certain hereditary examples may make a few people bound to get RA than others.

How Can It Affect Your Body?

Immune framework cells move from the blood into your joints and the tissue that lines them. This is known as the synovium. When the cells show up, they create inflammation. This causes your joints to swell as liquid develops to inside it. Your joints become painful, swollen, and warm to the touch.

After some time, the inflammation wears out the ligament, a comfortable layer of tissue that covers the parts of the bargains as you lose ligament, the space between your bones limits. Over the long haul, they could rub against one another or move strangely. The cells that cause inflammation additionally make substances that damage your bones.

The inflammation in RA can spread and influence organs and frameworks all through your body, from your eyes to your heart, lungs, kidneys, veins, and even your skin.
Blood Tests

Notwithstanding checking for joint issues, your primary care physician will likewise blood tests to analyze RA. She'll be searching for:

Iron deficiency: People with rheumatoid joint inflammation may have a low number of red platelets.

C-responsive protein (CRP): High levels are likewise signs of inflammation.

A few people with rheumatoid joint inflammation may likewise have a constructive antinuclear antibody test (ANA), which demonstrates an autoimmune infection. However, the test doesn't indicate which autoimmune ailment.

Cyclic citrulline antibody test (anti-CCP): This increasingly explicit test checks for anti-CCP antibodies, which propose you may have a progressively forceful type of rheumatoid joint pain.

Erythrocyte sedimentation rate (ESR): How quick your blood clusters up in the base of a test tube appears there might be inflammation in your framework.

Rheumatoid factor (RF): Most, yet not all, individuals with rheumatoid joint pain have this antibody in their blood. Be that as it may, it can appear in individuals who don't have RA.

Rheumatoid Arthritis Treatment

Treatments incorporate medications, rest, work out, and, at times, a medical procedure to address joint damage.

Your choices will rely upon a few things, including your age, generally speaking, wellbeing, clinical history, and how serious your case is.

Medications

Numerous rheumatoid joint pain medications can ease joint pain, growing, and inflammation. A portion of these drugs forestalls or hinder the malady.

Drugs that straightforwardness joint pain and firmness include:

- Anti-fiery painkillers, similar to anti-inflammatory medicine, ibuprofen, or naproxen

- Pain relievers that you rub on your skin

- Corticosteroids, similar to prednisone

- Narcotic pain relievers

Your primary care physician may likewise give you solid medications called sickness, adjusting antirheumatic drugs (DMARDs). They work by meddling with or smothering your immune framework's attack on your joints.

Conventional DMARDs are frequently the principal line treatment for RA:

- Hydroxychloroquine (Plaquenil), which was created to treat jungle fever

- Methotrexate (Rheumatrex, Trexall), which was first evolved to treat malignancy

- Leflunomide (Arava)

- Sulfasalazine (Azulfidine)

Biologic reaction modifiers are man-made forms of proteins in human qualities. They're an alternative if your RA is progressively extreme, or if DMARDs didn't help. You may even take a biologic and a DMARD together. The specialist could likewise give you a biosimilar. These new drugs are close, precise of biologics that cost less. Biologics endorsed for RA include:

- Abatacept (Orencia),

- Adalimumab (Humira), adalimumab-atto (Amjevita)

- Anakinra (Kineret)

- Baricitinib (Olumiant)

- Certolizumab (Cimzia)

- Etanercept (Enbrel), etanercept-szzs (Erelzi)

- Golimumab (Simponi, Simponi Aria)

- Infliximab (Remicade), infliximab-dyyb (Inflectra)

- Rituximab (Rituxan)

- Sarilumab (Kevzara)

- Tocilizumab (Actemra)

- Tofacitinib (Xeljanz)

- Upadacitinib (Rinvoq)

Why Are Rest and Exercise Important for RA?

You should be dynamic. However, you likewise need to take on a steady speed. During flare-ups, when inflammation deteriorates, it's ideal for resting your joints. Utilizing a stick or joint supports can help.

At the point when the inflammation facilitates, it's a smart thought to work out. It'll keep your joints adaptable and reinforce the muscles that encompass them. Low-sway exercises, as energetic strolling or swimming, and delicate extending can help. You might need to work with a physical advisor from the start.

When Is Surgery Needed?

At the point when joint damage from rheumatoid joint inflammation has gotten serious, the medical procedure may help.

Is There a Cure?

In spite of the fact that there isn't a solution for rheumatoid joint pain, early, forceful treatment will help forestall inability and increment your odds of abatement.

5. PERIODONTITIS

What is periodontitis? The periodontal malady, ordinarily called gum illness, is a chronic and dynamic incendiary condition influencing the tissues encompassing and supporting the teeth (gingiva, periodontal tendons, and alveolar jawbone).

In the beginning period, the oral pathology is called gum disease, gums get swollen, redness shows up, and the delicate tissue may effectively bleedwhile brushing and flossing. The further developed and serious type of periodontal illness is known as periodontitis.

Right now, gums are not appended to the teeth surfaces they used to be, profound periodontal pockets structures, the alveolar bone begins to reabsorb, and dental components turn out to be free and fall regardless of whether they are healthy.

Among periodontitis causes, poor oral cleanliness is the most repeating. Microorganisms contained in the dental plaque aggravate the gingival tissue around the teeth. Periodontal ailment shows up with its initial side effects: growing, gum dying, redness, and sore.

Fundamental conditions, for example, HIV/AIDS, diabetes, osteoporosis, and weight, may likewise be considered periodontal sickness causes.

Most normal periodontitis chance elements include smoking, hereditary inclination, nutrients insufficiency, and certain medications.

As announced by The American Academy of Periodontology right now of American grown-ups (pretty much 64.7 million individuals), endure as a result of mellow, moderate or propelled periodontitis, the further developed phase of periodontal malady that prompts teeth misfortune

In grown-ups, 65 years of age and more established, things deteriorate in certainty the rate significantly expands, arriving at 70.1%.

Periodontitis are diagnosed by a periodontist through a full periodontal assessment. Visual examination of gingival tells the clinician how healthy your gums are. X-beams test permits the specialist to assess the bone ingestion grade.

To wrap things up, periodontal testing and graphing give the periodontist the specific gum pockets profundities around a tooth. After all these diagnosis strategies, the expert can undoubtedly assess the condition of the strength of the teeth supporting structures.

Therefore, the periodontitis treatment requires a full periodontal examination first and the expert teeth cleaning by the dental specialist or dental hygienist. Scaling and root planing have the extension to expel tainted tissue from the tooth surface and from gum pockets. In the most serious cases, so as to finish the periodontal therapy, antibiotics, and oral medical procedure speak to the final hotel to dispose of periodontitis.

3 periodontal infection stages and pathology movement

Healthy gums

As appeared by the picture above, healthy gums are light pink and consummately appended to the tooth surface. The gingival sulcus depth(or gingival section) is around 1 to 3 mm. There is no dental plaque and no analytics (tartar) around teeth or underneath the gum line. Gums don't drain and don't hurt.

Periodontal sickness organize 1: mellow periodontitis definition

At its beginning time, parodontopathy is generally known as gum disease in light of the fact that the inflammation influences the gingival tissue just that gets red. The gums will start to be pulling away from the tooth, leaving an all the more profound gingival sulcus (3 to 5 mm).

The gum pockets (the space between the tooth cementum and the gingiva) shape and get further step by step if left untreated.

At the point when you brush and floss your teeth, you may likewise observe a couple of drops of blood blended in with the toothpaste and the water.

Because of the dental plaque and tartar aggregation, moderate awful breath or halitosis shows up.

Right now organize, the disease doesn't influence the alveolar bone yet, so teeth are as yet steady and can bolster the bite pressure. Gentle periodontitis is a reversible pathology implying that the dental specialist can without much of a stretch recuperate your gums.

Gentle periodontitis treatment includes proficient teeth and gums cleaning by the dental specialist or the dental hygienist and a satisfactory everyday oral consideration at home. Antiseptic mouthwashes, for example, oral washes with chlorhexidine gluconate, are viable to monitor microbes and periodontal inflammation.

Periodontal malady organize 2: moderate periodontitis definition

The second phase of the parodontopathy adds progressively serious periodontitis side effects to those recorded previously. Periodontal pockets are all the more profound, 5 to 7 mm. Gum downturn leaves the tooth root revealed, and teeth show up longer.

The periodontal Inflammation attacks the supporting bone, and 30% to half of the jawbone is lost (clinical connection misfortune).
Due to the underlying bone resorption, teeth begin to turn out to be somewhat free. The awful breath increments, and you will feel an unsavory preference for your mouth.

The dental specialist can just play out the treatment of moderate periodontitis. The clinician needs to evacuate the necrotic tissue brought about by the microbes contamination first. The excited region needs a few arrangements to return to the typical condition just as circumspect every day oral cleanliness at home.

Periodontal illness organize 3: propelled periodontitis definition

The third phase of periodontitis is the last one preceding the tooth misfortune, the most forceful and the hardest to treat.

Generally, dental specialists state that this periodontal sickness type isn't reversible, implying that it is conceivable to diminish the gingival inflammation; however, not to expel it totally.

Forceful periodontitis indications incorporate periodontal pockets further than 7 mm. The Infection arrives at the tip of the tooth root (summit). Terrible breath gets chronic, and the bone misfortune is around half (clinical connection misfortune). Now teeth don't have sufficient bone help and are close to falling unexpectedly.

Forceful periodontitis treatment may require laser therapy so as to murder whatever number microscopic organisms as could reasonably be expected. Gum medical procedure Is the final retreat to attempt to recuperate or supplant the tainted tissue.

Early signs and periodontitis indications

In the beginning times, periodontitis has not very many side effects. What is the reason it is designated "the quiet sickness."

Since gingival pain isn't the most widely recognized sign, inflammation may advance essentially before patients search for dental specialist help.

Early signs may include:

- Modest gum seeping in the wake of brushing and/or flossing;

- Change in the gums shading from pink to red (gingival redness) due to the periodontal inflammation;

- Slight gum growing;

- Moderate halitosis (bad breath);

- Change in taste view of foods.

- Propelled periodontitis indications:

- Gum draining is increasingly incessant, and it happens even without a trigger reason (precipitously);

- Important gum downturn that leaves revealed the cementum of the tooth, which is progressively touchy to plaque amassing and to the activity of the microscopic organism. In view of the gum downturn, teeth may show up longer than expected;

- The deep gum pockets between the teeth surface and gums;

- Persistent awful breath and metallic preference for the mouth;

- Loose teeth: this is the aftereffect of the dynamic supporting bone devastation brought about by the bacterial inflammation;

- vertical bone misfortune;

- bite change (the connection between the upper and lower teeth when they meet up shutting the mouth or biting food);

- partial of full false teeth don't accommodate your gums impeccably as they used to do;

- swollen face;

- ear and neck pain;

- jaw pain;

- fever;

- Swollen neck lymph hubs.

Periodontitis normal treatment and home cures

Sustenance assumes a basic job in keeping our whole creature in great condition, and this additionally applies to the mouth. A fair diet, plentiful in nutrients and minerals just as low in sugar, assists with keeping an oral hole and gums pathologies away.

Close by customary drugs therapy, and there are viable normal cures that can diminish the side effects of periodontal sickness and advance recuperating. Among them we can discover:

Coenzyme Q10 for periodontal infection

From its revelation (1957) until this point in time, inquires about and clinical investigations have demonstrated that Coenzyme Q10 assumes a crucial job in the treatment of diseases influencing human tissues, for example, gum disease and parodontopathy.

Our liver can incorporate this coenzyme from substances, for example, lipids and proteins.

As we age, this capacity diminishes; hence it is essential to take dietary enhancements or pick food containing it. Red meat, fish, regular natural products (apples, strawberries, and oranges) are generally wealthy in Coenzyme Q10 (CoQ10).

The primary coenzyme Q10 features are:

- It reinforces the immune framework and makes it more grounded in battling periodontal contamination;

- It is an incredible antioxidant viable against free radicals;

- Contributes to the periodontal tissue normal substitution.

Nutrient D and calcium to treat periodontitis

Calcium and Vitamin D (likewise called the Sunshine Vitamin) are essential for the upkeep of our bones, maxilla, and mandible notwithstanding. More grounded bones can all the more likely oppose to periodontal contamination that causes diseases influencing the gingival tissue. If there is an occurrence of Vitamin D inadequacy, there are extraordinary enhancements sold at drug stores or homegrown shops.

Aloe Vera: common periodontal infection treatment

Aloe Vera is a topical periodontitis common cure. Made out of numerous substances including cinnamic corrosive, Aloe Vera is notable for its anti-provocative, calming, and recuperating activity. Patients can utilize Aloe Vera gel legitimately on the aroused gums to get quick alleviation.

Propolis: periodontitis home cure

Normal cure with antibacterial and anti-fiery properties.

The tea Tree essential oil.

The tea tree oil (essential oil) is the best normal cure if there should arise an occurrence of periodontitis. A couple of drops of tea tree essential oil are sufficient to quiet down the excited tissues around the teeth

Periodontitis causes and hazard factors.

The Periodontitis is the inflammation of the periodontal structures that keep every tooth set up. The clinical term is periodontium that is made by:

1. Gingival tissue additionally called gum tissue;

2. Cementum: the outside surface of the teeth roots,

3. Alveolar bone: the attachments where, in typical condition, dental components are kept into

4. Periodontal tendons (PDLs) are filaments made of connective tissue that truly associate the tooth root to the alveolar bone.

Since we know which anatomic structures are associated with keeping up teeth in their position, it is all the more straightforward how periodontitis prompts bone misfortune and teeth to fall. Instrument

The essential driver of periodontitis is the bacterial plaque. Plaque is an imperceptible and clingy biofilm that holds fast to the gums and teeth. The plaque microscopic organisms produce toxins that arouse gums and disintegrate teeth finish.

If not expelled, the plaque solidifies (particularly beneath the gum line) and becomes tartar (math), which can't be evacuated just by utilizing the toothbrush. The tartar takes care of the periodontal inflammation that slips into the gingival pockets to find a good pace. At the point when gum disease advances to periodontitis, the contamination makes the bone reabsorb, and teeth stay without the important hard help and fall.

Among periodontitis causes, microbial plaque collection is essential; however, by all accounts, not the only one reason. Truth be told, there are a few extra periodontal sicknesses causes that may incorporate foundational conditions and terrible practices as depicted underneath.

Hereditary helplessness and genetic elements

Various examinations uncover that 30% of the total populace acquire the hereditary weakness to create periodontal sickness. The genetic elements clarify the motivation behind why even individuals who practice great oral cleanliness endure due to gum disease that progresses to periodontitis.

Insufficient dental rebuilding efforts, supports, and halfway false teeth

Orthodontic supports increment the danger of gum disease and chronic periodontitis since metal or plastic sections, metal groups, and curve wire offer to the plaque many concealing spots. Brushing and flossing while at the same time, wearing orthodontic supports, is a pain.

Sections make it hard to totally expel food flotsam and jetsam from your teeth. The plaque left between sections can trigger the disease that causes periodontal inflammation, draining, and growing. Grown-ups and youngsters with orthodontic supports should give more consideration to their dental cleanliness.

Fractional false teeth, dental scaffold, and inadequate prosthetic reclamation (dental crown, tooth filling) may likewise cause microbial plaque maintenance. If this occurs, it is strongly prescribed to request that your dental specialist fix the issue.

Unfortunate propensities: smoke and liquor misuse

Smoking is one of the primary periodontitis hazard factors. Truth be told inquires about uncover that odds of creating periodontitis are considerably more high in smokers than in non-smokers.

The nicotine contained in the cigarettes is a vasoconstrictor, implying that it makes the veins shrivel. The fundamental outcome of more tightly veins is that gingival tissue gets considerably less oxygen and white platelets. Presently it is anything but difficult to figure the motivation behind why inflammation can advance all the more effectively: basically in light of the fact that microscopic organisms find fewer adversaries.

Likewise, periodontitis treatment is less powerful in smokers than in individuals who never smoked cigarettes throughout their life because of the less fortunate recuperating.

Lack of healthy sustenance and Vitamins inadequacy

Among the reasons for periodontitis, we ought to likewise incorporate a lack of healthy sustenance that is the outcome of non-ideal living conditions, as in some less evolved nations.

Nutrients insufficiency happens when the diet is poor in minerals and nutrients that are vital for our body.

Periodontitis connected to foundational conditions

Heart diseases and strokes

Periodontal inflammation and gum malady can build the danger of coronary illness and stroke. Studies and research have demonstrated that microscopic organisms answerable for periodontitis can enter the circulatory system and arrive at the heart.

The oral microscopic organisms open the patient to create blood clumps, expanding the likelihood of stroke.

Osteoporosis and tooth misfortune

The teeth misfortune in patients influenced by osteoporosis and periodontitis is quicker in light of the fact that osteoporosis diminishes the jawbone thickness, and parodontopathy annihilates the bone itself. Teeth stay without the vital help structure and fall.

Periodontal ailment and diabetes

The periodontal disease makes it progressively hard to control glucose levels.

This happens in light of the fact that contamination in any piece of the body builds the measure of sugar in the blood. So diabetics need a bigger portion of insulin to balance. Periodontal inflammation likewise makes blood glucose levels increasingly hard to control.

Stress and immunosuppressive conditions

Consistently our immune guards shield us from a wide assortment of possibly dangerous microorganisms.

The human body can battle dangerous microscopic organisms and infections on account of the immune guards created during social advancement and adjustment to nature.

In any case, when the body is under pressure, our protections are brought down, microscopic organisms show signs of improvement and start their pathogenic activity.

At the level of the gum, inflammation will, in general, increment because of stress, permitting microscopic organisms to cause gum disease that progress to periodontal sickness.

Immunosuppressive conditions, for example, HIV/AIDS and leukemia lower, the immune framework advancing the movement of gingival tissue inflammation to periodontitis.

Periodontitis during pregnancy

Factual investigations have affirmed that pregnant ladies with periodontal issues are considerably more liable to bring forth untimely infants than ladies with healthy gums.

Past that, periodontitis during pregnancy appears to constrain the development of fetal development in the mother's belly. The child is bound to be brought into the world underweight.

Periodontal malady diagnosis by the periodontist

The periodontal malady diagnosis is made by a dental specialist who had practical experience in periodontics. The periodontal assessment comprises two principal parts: the first is the visual/mechanical evaluation of the patient's oral condition.

The clinician continues searching for gum pockets and, assuming any, and it is important to quantify their profundity and record the position creating a graph. The periodontal outlining is helpful to check the gum infection movement or mending.

During the visual evaluation, the periodontist will likewise search for free or moving teeth.

The second step of the periodontal assessment is made by the x-beams test and hereditary test.

How is periodontitis treatment?

After the periodontal visit and taking x-beams, the periodontist continues with the initial step of the parodontopathy therapy that includes the expert teeth cleaning by the dental specialist or dental hygienist.

Proficient cleaning

Freely from periodontal ailment organizes, the principal method to fix the parodontopathy requires the expert cleaning of every tooth surface (masticatory included). The clinician or the hygienist will utilize manual or potentially ultrasonic instruments to evacuate; however, much plaque as could be expected to diminish the contamination source.

Scaling or curettage and root planning

At the point when the dental specialist identifies solidified plaque beneath the gum line, at that point, particular dental cleaning instruments called curettes or scalers are required to expel hard tartar stores from the tooth root.

The root planning the methodology the periodontist uses to smooth the foundations of the teeth and evacuate all the necrotic gingival tissues and the periodontal contamination.

Teeth cleaning

After plaque and tartar stores expelling, the dental specialist will utilize extraordinary glue and sticky cups to clean your teeth roots and crowns. Actually, a smooth surface can confine or postpone the microbial biofilm where bacterial disease begins.

Antibiotic therapy

In the wake of cleaning the pockets, it is important to keep them clean and purified. For this reason, the dental specialist puts exceptionally little coagulated folds containing an antibiotic called doxycycline, which is discharged gradually.

Notwithstanding nearby antibiotics, your periodontist may recommend a turn of foundational antibiotics, for example, Amoxicillin (oral tablet or case), to battle the chronic periodontitis, which progressively hard to fix because of the contamination obstruction.

Periodontal medical procedure

On the off chance that non-careful therapy doesn't permit to arrive at the normal mending result, periodontal medical procedure speaks to the last opportunity to stop the movement of the inflammation and the loss of the bone. What's more, the periodontal medical procedure fundamental degree is to recover lost bone where conceivable.

There is a diverse periodontal medical procedure methodology:

- Open fold debridement

- Gum Grafts

- Bone uniting

Periodontitis laser therapy

Periodontitis laser therapy is an integral and moderately new dental methodology to fix periodontal infection without medical procedure. The laser can undoubtedly focus on the contaminated gingival tissue and consume it without doing any damage to the regular encompassing structures.

Furthermore, the laser can advance the tissue and bone recovery just as stop the gum draining very quickly since the main treatment.

Periodontal ailment laser therapy is less obtrusive than the oral medical procedure, and the recuperation is quicker.

Support and customary subsequent meet-ups

Periodontal ailment is a troublesome pathology to annihilate thusly the best outcome accompanying dental specialist treatments and day by day oral cleanliness support at home by the patient.

Standard subsequent meet-ups permit the specialist to monitor the inflammation and assess the mending procedure. Ordinary subsequent meet-ups additionally permit your dental specialist to find ahead of time new inflammation locales and treat them in their beginning time.

Is periodontal illness infectious?

The past inquiry just as the accompanying "Would periodontitis be able to be passed on by kissing or sharing a toothbrush ?" are the more asked by patients.

The inflammation is the sign our body is attempting to battle the disease.

That being stated, it is conceivable to spread microbes causing the periodontitis contamination through spit.

If there should be an occurrence of you know at least one your relatives endure as a result of parodontopathy, it is constantly prescribed not to share eating devices, for example, fork or spoon. To maintain a strategic distance from microscopic organisms to spread through spit, it is better not to share oral wellbeing hardware, for example, the toothbrush.

Step by step instructions to forestall periodontitis

You can forestall periodontal inflammation and stop the movement of gum disease to periodontitis by receiving sufficient oral cleanliness habits. The great oral consideration additionally requires visiting your dental specialist two times every year for proficient teeth cleaning and full mouth assessment.

As referenced toward the start of the book, microscopic organisms are the primary gum disease cause, particularly when microbial plaque amasses underneath the gumline. If not expelled, dental plaque mineralizes turning out to be hard analytics stores (tartar).

There are a couple of straightforward; however, significant standards to follow so as to forestall gum disease to create to periodontal sickness; some of them are recorded beneath:

Periodontal infection avoidance thusly starts at home, rehearsing the most precise oral cleanliness as would be prudent.

Brushing

Dental specialists consistently guidance patients to brush in any event multiple times after every meal (lunch and supper). One moment for every dental curve is sufficient. Recall not to utilize toothbrushes with hard fibers since you may incidentally damage your gums and make them drain.

Dental floss, interdental brushes, and floss picks

Little spaces in the middle of teeth are hard to keep clean. Flossing with customary dental string encourages you to evacuate more plaque close to the papilla and under the gumline. On the off chance that the hole between your teeth is enormous, interdental brushes are the correct devices to finish the oral cleanliness practice.

Floss picks are all the more simple to use for youngsters and individuals with huge fingers. Make sure to give more consideration cleaning around rooked or swarmed teeth, underneath dental scaffolds, and the obvious surface of fractional affected intelligence teeth.

Pick the fitting mouthwash.

The mouthwash is imperative to battle microbes in your mouth, so periodontists guidance their patients to utilize an antibacterial mouthwash with chlorhexidine gluconate (0.2% least).

Rotating brush and WaterPik

A few tests have exhibited that utilizing an electric toothbrush is conceivable to effectively expel more plaque than utilizing a manual one. The explanation is that the toothbrush head can move in various ways cleaning all the more profoundly.

WaterPik has demonstrated helpful and successful in expelling food trash from between dental components, props, and sections.

Keep away from clingy food and sugary drinks.

Acidic or clingy food just as game sugar drinks create an acidic oral condition where microscopic organisms can without much of a stretch multiply and develop in number. The consequence of the uneven proportion between all microorganisms that live in our mouth is gum inflammation.

5. ULCERATIVE COLITIS AND CROHN'S DISEASES

WHAT IS ULCERATIVE COLITIS

Ulcerative Colitis is a condition which causes inflammation and ulceration of the inward covering of the colon and rectum (the huge inside). Inflammation is the body's response to aggravation, injury or contamination, and can cause redness, expanding, and pain. In Colitis, ulcers create on the outside of the inside coating, and these may drain and produce bodily fluid.

The inflammation typically starts in the rectum and lower colon, however, it might influence the whole colon. In the event that Colitis just influences the rectum, it is called proctitis.

Ulcerative Colitis is one of the two principal types of Inflammatory Bowel Disease, so it may likewise be called 'IBD.' The other principal type of IBD is a condition known as Crohn's Disease.

Colitis is once in a while portrayed as a chronic condition. This implies it is progressing and deep-rooted, despite the fact that you may have extensive stretches of good wellbeing known as reduction, too backslides, or flare-ups when your side effects are progressively dynamic. Everybody is unique – in numerous individuals, the malady is gentle with scarcely any flare-ups, while others may have a progressively extreme ailment.

At present, there is no solution for Ulcerative Colitis. However, drugs, and once in an awhile medical procedure, can give significant stretches of alleviation from indications. Research, including work supported by Crohn's and Colitis UK, is proceeding into new treatments to improve patients' personal satisfaction and, in the end, discover a fix.

Side effects

Ulcerative Colitis side effects may run from gentle to serious and shift from individual to individual.

They may likewise change after some time, with times of abatement where you have great wellbeing and no side effects, substituting with backslides or flare-ups when your manifestations are inconvenient.

Colitis is an extremely singular condition - a few people can stay well for quite a while, in any event, for a long time, while others have visit flare-ups.

Your side effects may shift as indicated by the amount of the colon is kindled and how serious the inflammation is, yet the most widely recognized manifestations during an erupt are:

Looseness of the bowels. This is frequently with blood and bodily fluid, and a dire need to race to the can

• Cramping pains in the midriff. These can be extreme and frequently happen before passing a stool.

• Tiredness and weakness. This can be because of the disease itself, from iron deficiency (see beneath), or from an absence of rest on the off chance that you need to keep finding a workable pace with pain or looseness of the bowels.

• Feeling commonly unwell. A few people may have a raised temperature and feel hot, with a quick heartbeat.

• Loss of hunger and loss of weight.

• Anemia (a reduced number of red platelets). You are bound to create sickliness on the off chance that you are losing a great deal of blood or not eating admirably. Iron deficiency can cause you to feel tired.

WHAT CAUSES ULCERATIVE COLITIS

In spite of the fact that there has been a lot of research, we, despite everything, don't know precisely what causes Ulcerative Colitis. Anyway, significant advances have been made in the course of recent years, especially in hereditary qualities.

Analysts currently accept that Ulcerative Colitis is brought about by a mix of components: The qualities an individual has acquired + a strange response of the immune framework + something activated in nature.

Infections, microbes, diet, and stress have all been recommended as natural triggers, yet there is no positive proof that any of these variables is the reason for Crohn's or Colitis.

HOW COMMON IS ULCERATIVE COLITIS

It is evaluated that Ulcerative Colitis influences around one in every 420 individuals in the UK.

Colitis is more typical in urban than provincial zones, and in northern created nations - despite the fact that the numbers are starting to increment in creating countries. Colitis is likewise progressively basic in white Europeans, particularly those of Ashkenazi Jewish plummet (the individuals who lived in Eastern Europe and Russia).

Colitis influences ladies and men similarly. It will, in general, grow all the more much of the time in individuals who don't smoke or used to smoke than current smokers. Be that as it may, wellbeing experts consider the dangers of smoking greatly exceed any advantages found in Colitis, and unequivocally dishearten smoking in anybody, regardless of whether they have IBD. For more subtleties, see our data on Smoking and IBD.

WHAT ARE MAIN TYPES OF ULCERATIVE COLITIS

Ulcerative Colitis is commonly ordered by the amount of the internal organ is influenced. The chart shows the three principal types: proctitis, left-sided or distal colitis, and complete or pancolitis.

Proctitis

In proctitis, just the rectum (the most minimal piece of the enormous entrail) is excited. This implies the remainder of the colon is unaffected can even now work ordinarily. For some individuals with proctitis, the primary indication is passing new blood or bloodstained bodily fluid. You may get looseness of the bowels, or you may have typical stools or even obstruction. You may likewise feel a critical need to hurry to the latrine. Since the aroused rectum is increasingly delicate, a few people with proctitis frequently feel that they have a desire to pass a stool. However, it can't pass anything as the entrail is really unfilled. This is called tenesmus.

In certain individuals, the sigmoid colon (the short bending bit of colon closest the rectum) may likewise be excited – a type of Colitis now and again known as proctosigmoiditis. The side effects are like those of proctitis, in spite of the fact that obstruction is more outlandish.

Left-sided (or Distal) Colitis

Right now, Colitis, the inflammation includes the distal colon, which incorporates the rectum and the left half of the colon (otherwise called the plummeting colon). Manifestations incorporate loose bowels with blood and bodily fluid, pain on the left half of the belly, criticalness, and tenesmus.

Complete Colitis/Pancolitis

Colitis that influences the whole colon is known as absolute colitis or pancolitis. In the event that the inflammation influences the greater part of the colon; however, not every last bit of it, it is known as broad.

Colitis. Broad and complete colitis can cause extremely visit looseness of the bowels with blood, bodily fluid, and once in awhile discharge (a thicker, more yellow liquid than bodily fluid). You may likewise have serious stomach spasms and pain, tenesmus, fever, and weight misfortune. In milder flare-ups, the primary side effect might be looseness of the bowels or looser stools without blood.

Can Ulcerative Colitis include inconveniences inside the gut?

In exceptionally uncommon cases, Ulcerative Colitis can cause extra issues in the gut. These difficulties include:

Strictures

A stricture is a narrowing of the inside brought about by continuous inflammation that can make it hard for dung (stool) to go through the colon. Strictures don't normally happen in Colitis, yet can some of the time be an indication of inside disease.

Punctures

Exceptionally dynamic inflammation in the inside divider or a serious blockage brought about by a stricture may every so often lead to an aperture (crack) of the gut. This makes a gap which the substance of the entrail can spill through. This is an uncommon health-related crisis, manifestations of which incorporate serious stomach pain, fever, sickness, and spewing.

Poisonous Megacolon

At the point when the inflammation is broad and extreme, stomach related gases may get caught in the colon, making it swell up. This is known as lethal megacolon, which can happen in up to one of every 40 individuals with Colitis. Side effects incorporate a high fever just as pain and delicacy in the belly. It is essential to get treatment rapidly for this condition, as the medical procedure might be fundamental.

Fistulas

Individuals with Colitis, specifically the individuals who have had a pocket medical procedure (see What about careful treatment), can, in uncommon conditions, create fistulas. A fistula is a strange channel or way interfacing one inner organ to another, or to the outside surface of the body. Most fistulas (additionally called fistulae if multiple) start in the mass of the digestive system and associated pieces of the inside to one another, the vagina, bladder, or skin (especially around the butt).

6. SINUSITIS

Sinus disease (sinusitis) definition and realities

- Sinusitis or sinus disease is inflammation of the air cavities within the entries of the nose.

- Sinusitis can be brought about by disease, hypersensitivities, and concoction or particulate aggravation of the sinuses.

- Most individuals don't spread sinus infections to others.

- Sinusitis might be named acute sinus contamination, subacute sinus disease, chronic sinus disease, tainted sinusitis, and noninfectious sinusitis.

- Sinusitis signs and side effects incorporate.

- sinus cerebral pain,

- facial delicacy,

- pressure or pain in the sinuses, in the ears and teeth,

- fever,

- cloudy stained nasal or postnasal seepage,

- the feeling of nasal stuffiness,

- sore throat,

- cough, and

- occasionally facial expanding.

Symptoms of bacterial sinus contamination incorporate.

- ✓ facial pain,

- ✓ pus-like nasal release, and

- ✓ symptoms that endure for longer than a week and that are not reacting to over-the-counter (OTC) nasal medications.

• Sinus contamination is commonly analyzed dependent on patient history and physical assessment.

• Bacterial sinusitis is generally treated with antibiotics. Early treatment of allergic sinusitis may forestall auxiliary bacterial sinus infections.

• Home solutions for sinusitis and sinus infections incorporate over-the-counter (OTC) medications, for example, acetaminophen (Tylenol and others), decongestants, and mucolytics. The nasal water system can be practiced with a Neti-pot or wash unit (nasal bidet).

- Rare contagious infections of the sinuses (for instance, zygomycosis) are health-related crises.

- Complications of a sinus disease that may create are meningitis, mind canker, osteomyelitis, and orbital cellulitis.

- There are no contagious antibodies accessible to forestall parasitic sinus infections.

Is a Sinus Infection Contagious?

By what means Will I Know Whether I Have a Sinus Infection?

Most specialists imagine that the vast majority don't transmit sinus infections with the exception of uncommon occasions, and presume that sinus infections are not infectious.

Sinus infections, for the most part, start with the manifestations of a cold (for instance, a runny nose, infrequent hack or potentially gentle fever), and afterward form into pain and weight in the sinus depressions. Around 7 to 10 days after introductory cold-like side effects, different manifestations build-up that proposes you may have a sinus disease. Sinus disease manifestations incorporate.

- a yellowish-greenish nasal release that may have a smell,

- bad breath,

- puffiness around the eyes,

- headaches,

- pressure in the sinuses, and

- Coughing.

What are the sinuses? What number do we have?

A sinus is an empty, air-filled hole. For the motivations behind this book, a sinus will allude to those empty depressions that are in the skull and associated with the nasal aviation route by a thin opening in the bone (ostium). Typically all sinuses are available to the nasal aviation route through an ostium. People have four sets of these depressions each alluded to as the:

1.   frontal sinus (in brow),

2.   maxillary sinus (behind cheeks),

3.   ethmoid sinuses (between the eyes), and

4.   sphenoid sinus (profound behind the ethmoids).

The four sets of sinuses are frequently portrayed as a unit and named the "paranasal sinuses." The cells of the inward coating of every sinus are bodily fluid discharging cells, epithelial cells, and a few cells that are a piece of the immune framework (macrophages, lymphocytes, and eosinophils).

Elements of the sinuses incorporate humidifying and warming motivated air, protection of encompassing structures (eyes, nerves), expanding voice reverberation, and cradles against facial injury. The sinuses decline the weight of the skull. On the off chance that the inflammation ruins the freedom of mucous or obstructs the regular ostium, the inflammation may advance into a bacterial disease.

18 signs and side effects of sinus contamination or sinusitis

There are numerous signs and side effects of sinusitis and sinus infections. Coming up next is an outline of prevalent ones (18 aggregate) that may happen. Most patients have a few signs and side effects simultaneously. Others may have a few manifestations that are irregular; most don't have all side effects without a moment's delay. The signs and side effects of sinus contamination or sinusitis incorporate the accompanying:

1. Headache because of weight in mostly or totally blocked sinuses. The pain may increment when the individual twists down.

2. Facial delicacy as well as growing when facial regions over sinus regions are contacted.

3. Pressure or pain because of bodily fluid going ahead sinus tissue or inflammation of sinuses.

4. Fever because of the inflammation of sinus tissues and contamination.

5. A shady, stained nasal seepage is regularly observed in bacterial sinus infections.

6. Congestion is an inclination of nasal stuffiness and happens with both irresistible and non-irresistible sinusitis.

7. Postnasal trickle is bodily fluid overproduction from sinusitis that streams to the throat and aggravates throat tissue.

8. Sore throat is inflammation of throat tissue by a postnasal trickle.

9. Cough is a reaction to postnasal trickle and body's endeavor to get out throat tissue aggravations.

10. Tooth pain brought about by pressure on encompassing nerves and tissues

11. Ear pain brought about by pressure on encompassing nerves and tissues

12. Eye pain brought about by pressure on encompassing nerves and tissues

13.   Fatigue because of fever, immune reaction or potentially hacking

14.   Bad breath generally is because of bacterial infections

15.   Itching/sniffling - In noninfectious sinusitis, another related hypersensitivity symptoms of tingling eyes and wheezing might be normal. However, it may include a portion of the indications recorded above for irresistible sinusitis.

16.   Nasal seepage, for the most part, is clear or whitish-hued in individuals with noninfectious sinusitis.

17.   Ulceration can happen with uncommon fulminant parasitic infections with forcefully characterized edges and a dark, necrotic focus in the nasal territory. Some parasitic infections cause dull, dark showing up exudates. This requires prompt clinical assessment.

18.   Multiple chronic (more than one to a quarter of a year) manifestations generally are an indication of subacute or chronic sinusitis

What is a sinus disease or sinusitis?

Inflammation of the air pits inside the sections of the nose (paranasal sinuses) is alluded to as sinusitis. Sinusitis can be brought about by contamination (sinus disease), yet in addition, it can be brought about by sensitivity and compound disturbance of the sinuses. Sinus contamination (irresistible sinusitis) happens when an infection, bacterium, or a parasite develops inside a sinus.

Sinusitis is one of the more typical conditions that can torment individuals for the duration of their lives. Sinusitis normally happens when ecological dust bothers the nasal entries, for example, with roughage fever. Sinusitis can likewise result from aggravations, for example, chemicals or the utilization of potential maltreatment of over-the-counter (OTC) nasal splashes, and unlawful substances that might be grunted or breathed in through the nose. Around 30 million grown-ups have "sinusitis." Colds vary from sinusitis and are just brought about by infections and last around seven to 10 days while sinusitis may have a wide range of causes (irresistible and non-irresistible), and typically last longer with progressively articulated and variable manifestations.

What causes sinus infections or sinusitis?

Sinus infections or sinusitis might be brought about by whatever meddles with wind stream into the sinuses and the waste of bodily fluid out of the sinuses. The sinus openings (ostea) might be obstructed by expanding the tissue lining and nearby nasal section tissue, for instance with

- common colds,

- allergies, and

- Tissue aggravations, for example, OTC nasal showers, cocaine, and tobacco smoke.

Different reasons for sinus infections or sinusitis

Tumors or developments likewise can obstruct the sinuses on the off chance that they are close to the sinus openings.

Parchedness, ailment, drying medications and absence of adequate dampness can cause sinusitis or sinus infection. The seepage of mucus from the sinuses can likewise be impeded by thickening of the mucous emissions, by a decline in hydration (water content) of the mucous welcomed on by malady (for instance, cystic fibrosis), drying medications (antihistamines), and absence of adequate mugginess noticeable all around. The epithelial cells have little hair-like filaments, called cilia, which move to and fro to enable the bodily fluid to move out of the sinuses. These little cilia might be damaged by numerous aggravations, particularly smoke. This can keep them from helping the bodily fluid is depleting from the sinuses, and accordingly brings about sinus infections or sinusitis.

Stagnated bodily fluid gives a situation to microorganisms, infections, and in certain conditions (for instance, AIDS or immunosuppressed individuals) organism, to develop inside the sinus cavities. What's more, the microorganisms themselves can start and worsen sinus blockage. The most generally contaminated sinuses are the maxillary and ethmoid sinuses.

Once in a while, immunodepression or casualties of numerous injuries in calamities, for example, tidal waves, storms, seismic tremors, or tornadoes, may breathe in parasites from the dirt or water. In the end, in a couple of days to longer than seven days, the growths can develop and slice off blood supply to practically any kind of tissue, particularly in the nose and eyes. These infections, albeit uncommon, are not kidding and can be fatal and require quick clinical and careful consideration. Despite the fact that the parasitic contamination may look like regular bacterial sinusitis at first, it is a malady named zygomycosis or mucormycosis.

What are the types of sinusitis and sinus infections?

Sinusitis might be ordered in a few different ways, in light of its span (acute, subacute, or chronic) and the kind of inflammation (either irresistible or noninfectious). The term rhinosinusitis is utilized to infer that both the nose and sinuses are included an is turning into the favored term over sinusitis.

- Acute sinus contamination (acute sinusitis or acute bacterial rhinosinusitis) as a rule keeps going under 3-5 days.

- Subacute sinus contamination endures one to a quarter of a year.

- Chronic sinus contamination is greater than a quarter of a year. Chronic sinusitis might be further sub-ordered into chronic sinusitis with or without nasal polyps, or hypersensitive contagious sinusitis.

- Recurrent sinusitis has a few sinusitis attacks each year.

There is no clinical agreement on the above timespans.

- Infected sinusitis, for the most part, is brought about by uncomplicated infection contamination. Less much of the time, bacterial development causes sinus disease, and parasitic sinus contamination is rare. Subacute and chronic types of sinus disease, as a rule, are the aftereffect of deficient treatment of an acute sinus contamination.

- Noninfectious sinusitis is brought about by aggravations and unfavorably susceptible conditions and follows a similar general course of events for acute, subacute, and chronic as irresistible sinusitis.

What tests analyze the reason for sinus infections and sinusitis?

Sinus disease is regularly analyzed dependent on the history and assessment of a specialist. Since plain X-beam investigations of the sinuses might be deluding and methodology, for example, CT and MRI filters, which are considerably more touchy in their capacity to analyze sinus contamination, are so costly and not accessible in many specialists' workplaces, most sinus infections are at first analyzed and treated dependent on clinical discoveries on assessment. These physical discoveries may include:

- redness and expanding of the nasal sections,

- purulent (discharge like) seepage from the nasal sections (the indication well on the way to clinically analyze sinus contamination),

- tenderness to percussion (tapping) over the cheeks or brow locale of the sinuses, and

- Swelling about the eyes and cheeks.

Infrequently, nasal emissions are analyzed for discharged cells that may help separate among irresistible and hypersensitive sinusitis. Irresistible sinusitis may show specific cells of contamination (polymorphonuclear cells), while unfavorably susceptible sinusitis may show particular white platelets of hypersensitivity (eosinophils). Doctors recommend antibiotics if the bacterial disease is suspected. Antibiotics are not viable against viral infections; numerous doctors at that point treat the side effects.

In the event that sinus contamination neglects to react to the underlying treatment recommended, at that point, more top to bottom examinations, for example, CT or MRI sweeps, might be performed. Ultrasound has been utilized to analyze sinus infections in pregnant ladies. However, it isn't as precise as a CT or MRI. Rhinoscopy or endoscopy, a methodology for legitimately glancing in the rear of the nasal sections with a little adaptable fiberoptic cylinder, might be utilized to straightforwardly take a gander at the sinus openings and check for blockage of these openings by either expanding or developments.

It might now and again be important to play out a needle desire (needle cut) of a sinus to get tainted material to culture to figure out what microorganism is really causing the sinus contamination. Societies of the nasal sections are infrequently useful in figuring out what microscopic organisms or growth is causing a sinus disease since the nasal entries are regularly typically colonized by non-tainting microorganisms. The needle cut methodology is normally done by an otolaryngologist when treatments have neglected to mitigate the ailment. The technique requires neighborhood sedation to limit any distress; a few patients require general sedation. The sinus is suctioned, the substance sent for culture and recoloring, and the sinus might be flushed with a saline arrangement. This is, in fact, the most exact approach to analyze irresistible sinusitis.

Moreover, both inflexible and adaptable endoscopy has been utilized to get symptomatic material from sinuses. These methodologies are generally done by an otolaryngologist under topical and nearby sedation. Every so often, there might be a need to steady the patient. A few agents recommend that endoscopy examples are practically identical to those acquired by needle cut.

Contagious infections are typically analyzed by such biopsy methodology and tissue expelled by a specialist, or by parasitic culture, and tiny recognizable proof by a microbiologist or pathologist prepared to distinguish growths. Unfavorably susceptible contagious sinusitis (accentuation on hypersensitive) is a fiery reaction to parasitic components in the sinus hole and is suspected dependent on certain CT imaging attributes, just like the history and physical test.

What are the difficulties of sinus disease or sinusitis?

While genuine complexities don't happen much of the time, it is workable for sinus contamination to cause an immediate augmentation of disease into the mind through a sinus divider, creating a hazardous crisis (for instance, meningitis or cerebrum boil). What's more, other nearby structures can get tainted and create issues, for example, osteomyelitis of bones in the skull and disease around the eye (orbital cellulitis). Once in a while, these infections (essentially bacterial and parasitic life forms) may cause death. The most defenseless people to complexities are patients with stifled immune frameworks, diabetes, and moderately once in a while from numerous injury wounds that may happen in catastrophic events.

7. ACTIVE HEPATITIS

What is hepatitis?

Hepatitis alludes to a fiery state of the liver. It's usually brought about by viral contamination, yet there are other potential reasons for hepatitis. These incorporate autoimmune hepatitis and hepatitis that happens as an optional aftereffect of medications, drugs, toxins, and liquor. Immune system hepatitis is an ailment that happens when your body makes antibodies against your liver tissue.

Your liver is arranged in the right upper region of your tummy. It performs many basic capacities that influence digestion all through your body, including:

- bile creation, which is essential to assimilation

- filtering of toxins from your body

- excretion of bilirubin (a result of separated red platelets), cholesterol, hormones, and drugs

- breakdown of sugars, fats, and proteins

- activation of enzymes, which are particular proteins essential to body capacities

- Storage of glycogen (a sort of sugar), minerals, and supplements (A, D, E, and K)

- combination of blood proteins, for instance, egg whites

- synthesis of coagulating factors

Treatment alternatives shift contingent upon which sort of hepatitis you have. You can forestall a few types of hepatitis through inoculations and way of life safety measures.

The 5 types of viral hepatitis

Viral infections of the liver that are named hepatitis incorporate hepatitis A, B, C, D, and E. An alternate infection is liable for each sort of virally transmitted hepatitis.

Hepatitis An is constantly an acute, transient infection, while hepatitis B, C, and D are well on the way to get progressing and chronic. Hepatitis E is normally acute; however, it can be especially hazardous in pregnant ladies.

Hepatitis A

Hepatitis An is brought about by contamination with hepatitis An infection (HAV). This kind of hepatitis is most usually transmitted by expending food or water polluted by dung from an individual contaminated with hepatitis A.

Hepatitis B

Hepatitis B is transmitted through contact with powerful body fluids, for instance, blood, vaginal outflows, or semen, containing the hepatitis B contamination (HBV). Infusion drug use, engaging in sexual relations with a contaminated accomplice or imparting razors to a tainted individual increment your danger of getting hepatitis B.

It's assessed by the CDCTrusted Source that 1.2 million individuals in the United States and 350 million individuals overall live with this chronic ailment.

Hepatitis C

Hepatitis C originates from the hepatitis C infection (HCV). The Hepatitis C is transmitted to another patient through direct contact with contaminated body liquids, ordinarily through infusion drug use, and through sexual contact.

Hepatitis D

Also called delta hepatitis, hepatitis D is a genuine liver infection brought about by the hepatitis D infection (HDV). HDV is contracted through direct contact with tainted blood. Hepatitis D is an uncommon kinds of hepatitis that just happens related to hepatitis B disease.

Hepatitis E

Hepatitis E is a waterborne illness brought about by the hepatitis E infection (HEV). Hepatitis E is, for the most part, found in territories with poor sanitation and commonly comes about because of ingesting fecal issue that taints the water supply. Example of hepatitis E have been accounted for in the Middle East, Central America, Asia, and Africa, as indicated by the CDCTrusted Source.

Reasons for noninfectious hepatitis

Liquor and different toxins

Exorbitant liquor utilization can cause liver damage and inflammation. This is, in some cases, alluded to as alcoholic hepatitis. The liquor legitimately harms the cells of your liver. After some time, it can do lasting damage and lead liver disappointment and cirrhosis, thickening, and scarring of the liver.

Other dangerous reasons for hepatitis incorporate abuse or overdose of medications and presentation to harms.

Autoimmune framework reaction

Now and again, the immune framework botches the liver. It causes inflammation that can extend from mellow to serious, frequently upsetting liver capacity. It's multiple times more typical in ladies than in men.

Basic manifestations of hepatitis.

If you have irresistible types of hepatitis that are chronic, similar to hepatitis B and C, you might not have manifestations to start with. Indications may not happen until the damage influences liver capacity.

Signs and indications of acute hepatitis show up rapidly. They include:

- fatigue

- flu-like indications

- dark pee

- pale stool

- abdominal pain

- loss of craving

- unexplained weight misfortune

- yellow skin and eyes, which might be signs of jaundice.

Chronic hepatitis develops gradually, so these signs and indications might be too inconspicuous to even consider noticing.

How hepatitis is analyzed

History and physical test

To analyze hepatitis, first, your primary care physician will take your history to decide any hazard factors you may have for irresistible or noninfectious hepatitis.

During a physical assessment, your PCP may push down delicately on your stomach area to check whether there's pain or delicacy. Your PCP may likewise feel to check whether your liver is augmented. In the event that your skin or eyes are yellow, your primary care physician will take note of this during the test.

Liver capacity tests

Liver capacity tests use blood tests to decide how to productively your liver functions. Strange aftereffects of these tests might be the main sign that there is an issue, particularly in the event that you don't give any indications on a physical test of liver sickness. Higher liver enzyme levels may demonstrate that your liver is pushed, damaged, or not working appropriately.

Other blood tests

If your liver capacity tests are unusual, your primary care physician will probably arrange different blood tests to recognize the wellspring of the issue. These tests can check for the infections that cause hepatitis. They can likewise be utilized to check for antibodies that are regular in conditions like autoimmune hepatitis.

Ultrasound

A stomach ultrasound utilizes ultrasound waves to create a picture of the organs inside your guts. This test permits your primary care physician to take a close at your liver and close by organs. It can uncover:

•   fluid in your midriff

•   liver damage or augmentation

- liver tumors

- abnormalities of your gallbladder

The pancreas appears on ultrasound pictures too. This may be a helpful test in deciding the reason for your irregular liver capacity.

Liver biopsy

A liver biopsy is an intrusive strategy that includes your primary care physician taking an instances of tissue from your liver. Commonly, an ultrasound is utilized to direct your primary care physician when taking the biopsy test.

This test permits your primary care physician to decide how contamination or inflammation has influenced your liver. It can likewise be utilized to test any zones in your liver that seem irregular.

How hepatitis is treated

Treatment choices are dictated by which kind of hepatitis you have and whether the disease is acute or chronic.

Hepatitis A.

Hepatitis A doesn't require treatment since it's a transient ailment. Bed rest might be prescribed if indications cause a great arrangement of inconvenience. On the off chance that you experience retching or lose bowels, follow your physician's instructions for hydration and sustenance.

Hepatitis An antibody is accessible to forestall this contamination. Most youngsters start inoculation between ages 12 and a year and a half. It's a progression of two immunizations. Inoculation for hepatitis An is additionally accessible for grown-ups and can be joined with the hepatitis B antibody.

Hepatitis B

Acute hepatitis B doesn't require explicit treatment.

The Chronic hepatitis B is treated with antiviral medications. This type of treatment can be expensive because it must proceed for a while or years. Treatment for chronic hepatitis B additionally requires standard clinical assessments and observing to decide whether the infection is reacting to treatment.

Hepatitis B can be forestalled with inoculation. The CDCTrusted Source suggests hepatitis B immunizations for all babies. The arrangement of three antibodies is regularly finished over the initial a half year of youth. The antibody is likewise suggested for all social insurance and clinical faculty.

Hepatitis C

Antiviral medications are utilized to treat both acute and chronic types of hepatitis C. Individuals who create chronic hepatitis C are regularly treated with a mix of antiviral drug treatments.

People who create cirrhosis (scarring of the liver) or liver sickness because of chronic hepatitis C might be a contender for a liver transplant.

As of now, there is no inoculation for hepatitis C.

Hepatitis D

No antiviral medications exist for the treatment of hepatitis D right now. As per a 2013 study trusted Source, a drug called alpha interferon can be utilized to treat hepatitis D, yet it just shows improvement in around 25 to 30% of individuals.

Hepatitis D can be treated by getting the immunization for hepatitis B, as a disease with hepatitis B is fundamental for hepatitis D to create.

Hepatitis E

At present, no particular clinical treatments are accessible to treat hepatitis E. Since the contamination is regularly acute, it commonly settles all alone. Individuals with this sort of contamination are frequently encouraged to get satisfactory rest, drink a lot of liquids, get enough supplements, and maintain a strategic distance from liquor. In any case, pregnant ladies who build up this contamination require close observation and care.

Autoimmune hepatitis.

Corticosteroids, which is similar to prednisone or budesonide, are critical in the early treatment of autoimmune hepatitis. They're viable in around 80 percent of individuals with this condition.

Azathioprine (Imuran), a drug that smothers the immune framework, is frequently remembered for treatment. It very well may be utilized with or without steroids.

Tips to forestall hepatitis

Cleanliness

Rehearsing great cleanliness is one key approach to abstain from contracting hepatitis An and E. In case you're making a trip to a creating nation, you ought to keep away from:

- local water

- ice

- raw or half-cooked shellfish and clams

- raw products of the soil

Hepatitis B, C, and D contracted through polluted blood can be forestalled by:

- not sharing drug needles

- not sharing razors

- not utilizing another person's toothbrush

- not contacting spilled blood

Hepatitis B & Hepatitis C can be contracted through sex and private sexual contact. Rehearsing safe sex by utilizing condoms and dental dams can help decline the danger of contamination. You can discover numerous alternatives accessible to buy on the web.

Antibodies

The utilization of antibodies is a significant key to forestalling hepatitis. Immunizations are accessible to forestall the advancement of hepatitis An and B. Specialists are right now creating immunizations against hepatitis C. An inoculation for hepatitis E exists in China. However, it isn't accessible in the United States.

Confusions of hepatitis

Chronic hepatitis B or C can frequently prompt progressively genuine medical issues. Since the infection influences the liver, individuals with chronic hepatitis B or C are in danger for:

- chronic liver illness

- cirrhosis

- liver malignant growth

At the point when your liver quits working regularly, liver disappointment can happen. Confusions of liver disappointment include:

- bleeding scatters

- a development of liquid in your stomach area, known as ascites

- increased circulatory strain in entrance veins that enter your liver, known as entryway hypertension
- kidney disappointment

- hepatic encephalopathy, which can include weakness, memory misfortune, and decreased mental capacities because of the development of toxins, similar to smelling salts, that influence cerebrum work

- hepatocellular carcinoma, which is a type of malignant liver growth

- death

Individuals with chronic hepatitis B and C are urged to stay away from liquor since it can quicken liver infection and disappointment. Certain enhancements and medications can likewise influence liver capacity. On the off chance that you have chronic hepatitis B or C, check with your primary care physician before taking any new medications.

DAY MEAL PLAN

The vast majority have some thought that various foods can cause inflammation — and exacerbate pain.

Be that as it may, they, despite everything, don't know precisely what they ought to eat to take out their pain.

How inappropriate foods cause pain and inflammation

In the event that you live with chronic pain — regardless of whether it's back pain, joint pain, sciatica, or some other sort of pain — you're living in a condition of chronic inflammation.

So it bodes well that in the event that you need to kill pain, you need to reduce inflammation.

What's more, in the event that we needed to limit the wellspring of your inflammation to a certain something, it would almost certainly be the foods you eat all the time.

The absolute most significant thing you MUST do to dispose of pain is to eat an anti-incendiary diet.

What's more, the greatest obstacle for the vast majority — even the individuals who WANT to begin an anti-incendiary diet — is knowing which foods have anti-fiery properties and which foods really cause inflammation.

To make things considerably progressively entangled, not every person has the equivalent "trigger foods" — foods that cause their pain to erupt.

Foods that battle inflammation

A healthy eating methodology that consolidates anti-incendiary foods is your initial move toward diminishing inflammation and carrying on with a sans pain life.

Furthermore, the reward is that consolidating anti-incendiary foods into your diet has medical advantages that go past, essentially diminishing inflammation.

Many have been appeared to assume a job in forestalling various chronic diseases, including malignant growth, diabetes, and coronary illness.

Rather than vegetable oils, pick coconut oil or olive oil.

Coconut oil originates from the beefy product of the coconut and is pressed with medical advantages.

Its anti-fiery properties are so extraordinary; it's even been appeared to stop the damage of joint inflammation and reduce joint inflammation indications. Saute vegetables and coconut oil in a nonstick skillet or even add a spoonful to your espresso for a morning treat.

This is regularly called "Impenetrable Coffee."

Like coconut oil, olive oil is a decent wellspring of healthy fats.

Among them is an unsaturated fat called oleic corrosive, which has not exclusively been appeared to reduce inflammation. However, a few investigations show that it might even positively affect qualities that are connected to the disease.

Less pain in less than seven days with the best anti-incendiary diet recipes

The more regularly you eat foods that battle inflammation, the better you will feel!

The anti-fiery diet can help ease joint pain and reduce inflammation.

As per the Arthritis Foundation, certain foods can help handle inflammation, reinforce bones, and lift the immune framework.

Following a particular anti-provocative meal plan can assist individuals with making delectable, nutritious food while assisting with monitoring their inflammation.

26 anti-fiery recipes

The anti-fiery diet contains a lot of prebiotics, fiber, antioxidants, and omega-3s. This implies a diet wealthy in vegetables, whole organic products, whole grains, vegetables, and greasy fish.

Peruse on for 26 anti-fiery recipes to go after breakfast, lunch, supper, and tidbits.

Breakfast

Start off the day with the accompanying nutritious anti-provocative recipes:

1. Oat porridge with berries

Oats with berries passes on high parts of prebiotics, cell reinforcements, and fiber.

Oats are high in a sort of fiber called beta-glucans. Beta-glucans are a critical prebiotic for the gut microorganisms Bifidobacterium, which may help decrease diabetes-related aggravation and heaviness.

Prebiotics help the sound gut microorganisms to flourish, which can help lessen aggravation.

Berries are high in cancer prevention agents, and blueberries are especially high in hostile to ignitable polyphenols called anthocyanins.

Dietary tip: Traditional rolled and steel-cut oats are higher in fiber than speedy oats.

2. Buckwheat and chia seed porridge

Buckwheat groats are without gluten and a great substitute for oats for individuals who are touchy to gluten.

Including chia seeds will help the invigorating omega-3 substance of this morning meal decision.

Omega-3s assistance reduces inflammation in the body, and research shows that they can improve joint delicacy and solidness in individuals with RA.

Chia seeds are additionally high in fiber and protein, which will keep individuals feeling full for more.

3. Buckwheat berry flapjacks

Buckwheat is additionally a decent wellspring of two key anti-incendiary polyphenols called quercetin and rutin.

Quercetin is an antioxidant, while rutin has anti-incendiary properties, which may help with joint inflammation.

In spite of its name, buckwheat isn't a grain. It is the seed of products of the soil sans gluten. Buckwheat is particularly famous in Japanese cooking.

Numerous wellbeing food markets and online stores sell buckwheat.

4. Fried eggs with turmeric

Eggs are a brilliant wellspring of protein, and the egg yolk contains nutrient D.

Nutrient D could constrain the procedure of inflammation because of its consequences for the immune framework. The report additionally noticed that individuals with RA had lower nutrient D levels than others considered.

Add turmeric to fried eggs for an additional anti-provocative lift. Turmeric is a wealthy in a compound called curcumin, can help oversee oxidative and fiery conditions.

5. Smoked salmon, poached eggs and avocado on toast

Salmon and avocado are both rich wellsprings of anti-incendiary omega-3 unsaturated fats.

Eating a lot of restorative unsaturated fats can likewise improve heart wellbeing and lower an individual's danger of cardiovascular sickness.

This generous breakfast is great for extremely dynamic days or end of the week informal breakfasts. For sans gluten choices, use sans gluten bread.

Anti-Inflammatory Diet Meal Plan Intro/RESET

The anti-incendiary diet meal plan is a basic, healthy meal plan to reset your body from oxidative pressure. In case you're scared by healthy eating or confounded by the word anti-fiery, these anti-provocative recipes are for you! Realize what foods help reduce inflammation and get heavenly recipes that are sans gluten, refined without sugar, and sans dairy well disposed to oblige it!

Consider this Anti-Inflammatory Diet Meal Plan an INTRO to anti-incendiary rich foods. A smaller than usual reset meal plan. Alright?

Of course, you may be somewhat sore from the start. However, your body is attempting to fix those muscles, making them more grounded! This accompanies appropriate rest, recuperation, and sustenance! This acute inflammation likewise applies to another way of life factors that cause oxidative pressure (a lopsidedness between the creation of free radicals and the body's capacity to FIGHT or detoxify these harming impacts through antioxidants).

Instances of oxidative pressure are:

- excessive sun introduction
- smoke
- emotional stress
- Lack of rest, and so on.

A little introduction is fine (and here and there unavoidable) as long as the body recoups. Bode well?

So you see, we're attempting to concentrate on recovering the body in balance. I figure the best thing we can accomplish (for the time being) is, to begin with, food. Foods that recuperate!

Tenderfoot's Guide to an Anti-Inflammatory Diet

• Start by including a portion of these anti-fiery rich SUPERFOODS into your diet. Reduce the utilization of prepared foods and gluten when all is said in done. Ideally, this meal plan will be a guide. Pick a couple of recipes, at that point turn. Don't hesitate to peruse my other gluten-free and dairy-free meal plans as well!

The recipes beneath center around SUPERFOOD (anti-incendiary foods) that can help reduce inflammation. They are plentiful in nutrients (antioxidants), minerals, essential unsaturated fats, prebiotic and solvent fiber, probiotics, and that's just the beginning! My expectation is that these recipes will give you vitality to recover that body in balance. Presently we simply need to concentrate on the other way of life factors. Oye! I feel ya, going on and on needlessly here.

Anti-Inflammatory Diet Meal Plan

These anti-incendiary recipes incorporate heavenly and healthy choices for:

• breakfast

• lunch

• main dish/supper

• drinks

• snacks/dessert

Anti-Inflammatory Breakfast Recipes

Coconut Flour Pancakes

These coconut flour flapjacks have a low sugar choice, are normally improved, grain-free, anti-fiery rich berry beating!

No-Bake Lemon Coconut Paleo Energy Bars

These paleo vitality bars additionally have a low sugar choice, grain-free, anti-fiery rich coconut, and lemon besting! Incidentally, the video is posted in our Cotter Crunch Lots of individuals discussing these bars!

Clingy Date Cake Nourishing Bowls

These clingy date cake yogurt bowls are improved with you got it, dates! Wealthy in filaments, iron, and protein. For lower-sugar choice, excluding the fixing. For sans dairy alternative, use coconut milk yogurt or chilled coconut cream.

Chai Spiced Chia Smoothie Bowls

Amending smoothie bowl (or smoothie cup on the off chance that you want to drink it) wealthy in anti-provocative flavors anti-oxidant rich chai tea! You can spoon (or drink) this smoothie bowl warm or cold. It's eminent!

Anti-Inflammatory Lunch and Main Dish Recipes

Spiralized Apple Kimchi Salad with Beef

Fast apple kimchi serving of mixed greens with sesame meat! This Asian roused spiralized apple plate of mixed greens formula makes a brisk and healthy kimchi substitute. Wealthy in iron, phytonutrients, protein, and fiber!

Salted Pineapple Baja Fish Tacos

The garnish to these omega-rich fish tacos says everything! That's right, and pickling foods help jelly supplements and flavor! Nutrients, for example, A, D, E, and K, are additionally continued during the pickling procedure For prebiotic vegetables that are normally aged (for example, garlic, onion, cabbage, and artichokes), pickling can help hold B Vitamins and great microscopic organisms!

You should utilize paleo tortillas for this formula. We love Seite Almond Flour Tortillas or making our own with Naan Bread.

Lemony Herb Socca Pizza

For a without dairy choice, preclude the cheddar and utilize nourishing yeast.

This Socca pizza is produced using garbanzo bean (chickpea) flour, a stone-ground grain-free flour high in fiber, plant-based protein, and made with whole garbanzo beans—natively constructed veggie-lover pesto and lots of healthy garnishes like herbs.

- Basil, tarragon, and oregano leaves – Contain oils that have an antioxidant impact.

- Arugula – Vitamin K

- Lemon – Vitamin C

Coconut Rice and Watermelon Salad Bowls

Watermelon serving of mixed greens bowls is the ideal supporting, gluten-free veggie-lover bowl. Coconut cream, jasmine rice, watermelon, and raisins consolidate to create an astounding combo of hydration, healthy fats, and invulnerability boosting Vitamin C!

Asian Zoodle Flu Buster Soup

Brisk Asian Zoodle Flu Buster Soup! This Asian propelled paleo zucchini noodle soup is light yet wealthy in anti-incendiary properties. The red cabbage and Asian soup include an increase in recuperating supplements Vegetarian and Vegan alternatives!

Rosemary Citrus One Pan Baked Salmon

This Rosemary Citrus Baked salmon is a healthy one-skillet meal prepared quickly! A whole 30 one-dish meal is plentiful in omega 3's (essential unsaturated fats), Vitamin C, and herbs like Rosemary that can help reduce inflammation, facilitate the pain, and secure your immune framework.

Detox Broccoli Salad without Mayo

Add unfenced simmered chicken to this plate of mixed greens to make a total meal. Simply portending a formula coming soon as well. SO scrumptious!

This is one stacked plate of mixed greens with detoxifying veggies like broccoli, spinach, and blueberries hurled in light and tart olive oil yogurt sauce. For a dairy-free alternative, use non-dairy yogurt or thicken coconut cream.

Anti-Inflammatory Diet Drinks + Snacks

Handcrafted Fruit Kvass with Mint.

This handcrafted Fruit kvass with berries, lime, and mint is a gluten-free form of a well known Russian matured beverage. Stacked with probiotics, it's a reviving, tart, bubbly beverage that you can make comfortable.

Crude Veggies with Homemade Vegan Ranch Dressing

This delectable dressing can be slathered on a plate of mixed greens, filled in as a veggie plunge, or dunked in your preferred fiery foods. Vegetarian, whole 30, and paleo cordial, this velvety without dairy farm dressing are produced using mixed cashews, nut milk, herbs, and oil.

Maple Sesame Quinoa Bars (Nut Free)

Maple Sesame Quinoa Bars make a flavorful veggie-lover breakfast bar or vitality bar. A combo of maple, sesame seed, gluten-free oats, sunflower seed margarine, and quinoa create a sweet and nutty taste without nuts. A whole-grain quinoa bar stuffed with plant-based protein and supplements.

HOW TO MAKE THIS A LIFESTYLE

7-Day Sample Menu for Anti-Inflammatory Diet Beginners

The accompanying example menu isn't one-size-fits-all. However, it offers some creative thoughts for adding anti-incendiary foods to your meals. In case you're dealing with a specific infection, for example, diabetes, you may have certain dietary needs that this meal plan doesn't address. Make certain to counsel your medicinal services group before rolling out any significant improvements to your eating habits.

Day 1

Breakfast Steel-cut oatmeal with fragmented almonds and blueberries, and some espresso

Lunch Chopped kale plate of mixed greens with chickpeas, beets, and pomegranate seeds hurled with an olive oil and lemon juice vinaigrette

Supper Anchovy, salmon, and tomato-beat pizza on a cauliflower covering

Nibble Small bunch of natively constructed trail blend in with unsalted nuts and raisins

Day 2

Breakfast Steel-cut oatmeal beat with pecans and cut strawberries, and some espresso

The Lunch Salmon sashimi with a side of broccoli, and a side of darker rice and ginger

Supper Ginger curry with whitefish, kale, grain, and a glass of red wine

Tidbit Sliced mango

Day 3

Breakfast Quinoa bowl with cut banana, blueberries, and a shower of almond spread, alongside some green tea

Lunch Arugula plate of mixed greens with tuna fish, flame-broiled peaches, and pecans

Supper Spinach plate of mixed greens with flame-broiled salmon and a side of dark-colored rice

Bite Frozen grapes

Day 4

Breakfast Kale and mushroom frittata, a large portion of a grapefruit, and some espresso

Lunch Grain bowl with dark colored rice, chickpeas, and sautéed bok choy

Supper Veggie burger on a whole-grain bun with a side of broiled Brussels grows.

Nibble Small bunch of unsalted blended nuts

Day 5

Breakfast Chia seed pudding, apple cuts with almond spread, and some green tea

Lunch Spinach plate of mixed greens with fish and destroyed carrots

Supper Red peppers loaded down with ground turkey, quinoa, chickpeas, and a glass of red wine.

Nibble Small bunch of unsalted almonds

Day 6

Breakfast Soy yogurt with new blueberries and some espresso

Lunch Quinoa bowl with sardines, tomatoes, dark beans, sautéed spinach, and avocado

Supper Salmon with lentils and a spinach plate of mixed greens

Nibble A square of dull chocolate and a little bunch of unsalted blended nuts

Day 7

Breakfast Peanut spread and banana sandwich, and some espresso

Lunch Smashed avocado and split cherry tomatoes over whole-grain toast, and a side of curds.

Supper Seitan with chime peppers, mushrooms, and broccoli sautéed in olive oil

Nibble Cherries

PREPARING FOR HEALTHY CHANGE AND TIPS ON FOLLOWING AN ANTI-INFLAMMATORY DIET

Tips on Following an Anti-Inflammatory Diet

- Eat five to nine servings of antioxidant-rich leafy foods every day.

- Limit your admission of foods high in omega-6 unsaturated fats while expanding your utilization of foods wealthy in omega-3 unsaturated fats (for example, flaxseed, pecans, and sleek fish like salmon, fish, mackerel, and herring).

- Replace red meat with more advantageous protein sources, for example, lean poultry, beans, fish, soy, and lentils.

- Instead of picking refined grains, settle on fiber-rich whole grains like oats, quinoa, dark colored rice, bread, and pasta that rundown a whole grain as the main fixing.

- Rather than flavoring your meals with salt, upgrade enhance with anti-provocative herbs like garlic, ginger, and turmeric.

5 Tips for Maintaining an Anti-Inflammatory Diet Lifestyle

Need assistance beginning? We've arranged a couple of our most supportive tips:

1. Meal prep. Throughout the end of the week, choose your meals for the week. It will be simpler to eat healthy for the whole week on the off chance that you have a plan set up.

2.   Write a shopping list. Set up a basic food item list before you step foot in the store. You'll be less enticed to purchase comfort foods and tidbits.

3.   Choose an assortment of organic products, veggies, and healthy fats. Having choices will shield you from getting exhausted. In addition, broadening your meals will give you a full scope of supplements.

4.   Keep healthy bites close by. You'll be more averse to go after chips and treats if a superior alternative is close by.

5.   Drink more water. Appropriate hydration helps your vitality level, cerebrum capacity, and general wellbeing.

HOW TO PREPARE FOR A HEALTHY CHANGE

25 Simple Tips to Make Your Diet Healthier

A healthy diet has been experimentally demonstrated to give various medical advantages, for example, diminishing your danger of a few chronic diseases and keeping your body healthy.

Be that as it may, rolling out significant improvements to your diet can, in some cases, appear to be overpowering.

Rather than rolling out enormous improvements, it might be smarter, to begin with, a couple of little ones.

This book talks about 25 little changes that can make a standard diet somewhat more advantageous.

1. Take it easy

The point at which what you eat influence the sum you eat, similarly as the way that you are so at risk to gain weight.

In all honesty, mulls over taking a gander at changed eating speeds show that brisk eaters are dependent upon 115% bound to be fat than moderate eaters.

Your hankering, the amount you eat, and how full you get is completely obliged by hormones. These hormones signal your psyche, regardless of whether you're anxious or full.

Notwithstanding, it takes around 20 minutes for your mind to get these messages, so eating all the more gradually would give your cerebrum the time it needs to see that you are full.

Studies have affirmed this, indicating eating gradually may reduce the number of calories you devour at meals and assist you with shedding pounds.

Eating gradually is likewise connected to progressively exhaustive biting, which has additionally been connected to all the more likely weight support.

Along these lines, basically by eating increasingly slow more frequently, you can reduce your danger of eating excessively and putting on abundant weight.

2. Pick Whole-Grain Bread — Not Refined

Without much stretch, make your diet somewhat more advantageous by picking whole grain bread instead of conventional refined-grain bread.

Rather than refined grains, which have been connected to numerous medical problems, whole grains have been connected to an assortment of medical advantages, including a reduced danger of type 2 diabetes, coronary illness, and malignancy.

They are likewise a decent wellspring of fiber, B nutrients, and a few minerals, for example, zinc, iron, magnesium, and manganese.

There are numerous assortments of whole-grain bread accessible, and a significant number of them even taste superior to refined bread.

Simply try to peruse the mark to guarantee that your bread is made with whole grains just, not a blend of whole and refined grains. It's additionally best that the bread contains whole seeds or grains.

3. Add Greek-Yogurt to Your Diet

Greek-yogurt (or Greek-style yogurt) is thicker and creamier than standard yogurt.

It has been stressed to evacuate its abundance whey, which is the watery piece of milk. The final product is a yogurt that is higher in fat and protein than normal yogurt.

Truth be told, it contains up to multiple times the measure of protein found in a similar measure of customary yogurt, or as much as 9 grams for every 100 grams.

Eating a decent wellspring of protein causes you to feel more full for more, helping you deal with your hunger and eat less calories by and large.

Besides, since Greek yogurt has been stressed, it contains less carbs and lactose than customary yogurt, making it appropriate for the individuals who follow a low-carb diet or are lactose prejudiced.

Basically, supplant a few bites or customary yogurt assortments with Greek yogurt for a heavy portion of protein and supplements.

Simply make a point to pick the non-seasoned assortments, as enhanced ones might be stuffed with included sugar and other unhealthy fixings.

4. Try not to Shop Without a List

There are two significant methodologies to utilize when you go shopping for food: make your shopping list early and don't go to the store hungry.

Not knowing precisely what you need prepares for drivé purchasing, while craving can additionally worsen your motivations.

By doing this and adhering to your rundown, you won't just purchase more advantageous things yet, in addition, set aside cash and have more beneficial foods around the house.

5. Eat Eggs, Preferably for Breakfast

Eggs are unfathomably healthy, particularly in the event that you eat them toward the beginning of the day.

They are wealthy in great protein and numerous essential supplements that individuals frequently don't get enough of, for example, choline.

When seeing investigations looking at different types of calorie-coordinated morning meals, eggs beat the competition.

Eating eggs in the first part of the day expands sentiments of totality. This has been appeared to make individuals devour less calories throughout the following 36 hours, which can be very useful for weight misfortune.

One examination in healthy and fit youngsters demonstrated that eggs caused fundamentally more totality, less yearning, and a lower want to eat, contrasted with a morning meal comprising of oat or croissants.

Indeed, the men who had eggs for breakfast consequently ate 270–470 less calories at lunch and supper buffets, contrasted with the individuals who ate different morning meals.

Along these lines, basically supplanting your present breakfast with eggs may bring about significant advantages for your wellbeing.

6. Increment Your Protein Intake

Protein is regularly alluded to as the lord of supplements, and it seems to have a few superpowers.

Because of its capacity to influence your appetite and satiety hormones, it's the most filling of the macronutrients.

One examination demonstrated that basically expanding protein admission from 15% to 30% of calories caused individuals to eat 441 less calories for every day without effectively confining their admission.

Also, protein encourages you to hold bulk, which decides the pace of your digestion. A high protein admission may expand the number of calories you consume by 80–100 every day.

This is particularly significant for forestalling the loss of bulk that can happen during weight misfortune and as you age.

Plan to add a wellspring of protein to every meal and bite. It will assist you with feeling more full for more, check yearnings, and make you less inclined to overeat.

Great wellsprings of protein incorporate dairy items, nuts, nutty spread, eggs, beans, and lean meat.

7. Drink Enough Water

Drinking enough water is significant for your wellbeing.

Numerous examinations have indicated that drinking water may profit weight misfortune, weight support, and even somewhat increment the number of calories you consume day by day.

Concentrates additionally show that drinking water before meals can reduce hunger and calorie consumption during the resulting meal in moderately aged and more seasoned grown-ups.

So, the most significant thing is to drink water rather than different refreshments. This may definitely reduce your sugar and calorie consumption.

All things considered than individuals who drink different refreshments.

8. Prepare or Roast Instead of Grilling or Frying

The manner in which you set up your food can radically change its consequences for your wellbeing.

Flame broiling, cooking, fricasseeing, and profound singing are on the whole well-known strategies for getting ready meat and fish.

Be that as it may, during these types of cooking techniques, a few possibly lethal mixes are shaped, for example, polycyclic fragrant hydrocarbons (PAHs), propelled glycation finished results (AGEs) and heterocyclic amines (HCAs).

These mixes have been connected to a few diseases, including malignant growth and coronary illness.

More beneficial cooking strategies incorporate heating, searing, stewing, slow-cooking, poaching, pressure cooking, stewing, and sous-vide.

These techniques don't advance the development of these destructive mixes and, in this manner, make your food more advantageous.

In any case, there is nothing to state you can't appreciate the infrequent flame broil or profound fry, yet attempt to utilize those strategies sparingly.

9. Take Omega-3 and Vitamin D Supplements

An amazing number of individuals around the globe are insufficient in nutrient D, including 42% of the US populace.

Nutrient D is a fat-dissolvable nutrient that is significant for bone wellbeing and the best possible capacity of your immune framework. Truth be told, each cell in your body has a receptor for nutrient D, demonstrating its significance.

Nutrient D is found in not many foods, yet greasy seafood, by and large, contains the most noteworthy sums.

Omega-3 unsaturated fats are another generally deficient with regards to supplement found in greasy seafood. They have numerous significant jobs in the body, including lessening inflammation, keeping up heart wellbeing, and advancing mind work.

The Western diet is commonly extremely high in omega-6 unsaturated fats, which advance inflammation and have been connected to numerous chronic diseases.

Omega-3s assistance battle this inflammation and keep the body in an increasingly adjusted state.

If you don't eat greasy seafood consistently, you ought to think about taking an enhancement. Omega-3s and nutrient D can frequently be discovered together in an enhancement.

10. Supplant Your Favorite "Inexpensive Food" Restaurant

Eating out doesn't need to include unhealthy foods.

Consider "redesigning" your preferred drive-through joint to one with more beneficial alternatives.

There are numerous healthy drive-through eateries and combination kitchens offering heavenly and healthy meals.

They may simply be a great substitution for your preferred burger or pizza joint. Likewise, you can, by, and large, get these meals at a good cost.

11. Attempt, in any event, One New Healthy Recipe Per Week

Choosing what to have for supper can be a consistent reason for dissatisfaction, which is the reason numerous individuals will, in general, utilize similar recipes over and over.

Odds are you've been cooking similar recipes on autopilot for quite a long time.

If these are healthy or unhealthy recipes, it's constantly healthy to take a stab at something new.

Plan to take a stab at making another healthy formula at any rate once every week. This can switch up your food and supplement admissions and ideally add new and healthy recipes to your everyday practice.

12. Pick Baked Potatoes Over French Fries

Potatoes are very filling and a typical side to numerous dishes.

So, the strategy where they're arranged to a great extent decides their wellbeing impacts.

First of all, 100 grams of heated potatoes contain 94 calories, while a similar measure of french fries contains more than three-fold the number or 319 calories.

Moreover, southern style french fries commonly contain destructive mixes, for example, aldehydes and trans fat.

Supplanting your french fries with prepared or bubbled potatoes is a great method to shave off calories and dodge these destructive mixes.

13. Eat Your Greens First

A decent method to guarantee that you eat your greens is to eat them as a starter.

Thusly, you will probably complete the entirety of your greens while you are the hungriest and be well-suited to eat less of other, maybe less healthy, parts of the meal.

This may lead you to eat less and more beneficial calories, generally speaking, which may bring about weight misfortune.

Besides, eating vegetables before a carb-rich meal has appeared to effectively affect glucose levels.

It hinders the speed at which carbs are assimilated into the circulatory system and may profit both short-and long haul glucose control in individuals with diabetes.

14. Eat Your Fruits Instead of Drinking Them

Organic products are healthy. They are stacked with water, fiber, nutrients, and antioxidants.

Studies have repeatedly connected eating natural products to a reduced danger of a few diseases, for example, coronary illness, diabetes, and malignant growth.

Since natural products contain fiber and different plant aggravates, their sugars are commonly processed gradually and don't cause significant spikes in glucose levels.

Notwithstanding, the equivalent doesn't have any significant bearing for organic product juices.

Many natural product juices aren't produced using a genuine organic product but instead concentrate and sugar. They may even contain a lot of sugar as a sugary soda.

Indeed, even genuine organic product juices come up short on the fiber, and biting opposition gave by whole natural products. This makes natural product squeeze substantially more liable to spike your glucose levels.

It additionally makes it too simple to even think about consuming a lot at a time.

15. Cook at Home More Often

Attempt to make a habit of cooking at home most evenings, instead of eating out.

For one, it's simpler on your financial limit.

Second, by cooking your food yourself, you'll know precisely what is in it. You won't need to ponder about any shrouded unhealthy or fatty fixings.

Additionally, by cooking enormous servings, you will likewise have remains for the following day, guaranteeing a healthy meal at that point, as well.

At last, cooking at home has been appeared to reduce the danger of unnecessary weight gain, particularly among kids.

16. Become More Active

Great nourishment and exercise regularly go connected at the hip.

Exercise has been appeared to improve your state of mind, just as diminishing sentiments of wretchedness, tension, and stress.

These are the specific sentiments that are destined to add to passionate and voraciously consuming food.

Besides fortifying your muscles and bones, exercise may assist you with shedding pounds, increment your vitality levels, reduce your danger of chronic diseases, and improve your rest.

Plan to do around 30 minutes of moderate to high-force practice every day, or basically take the stairs and go on short strolls at whatever point conceivable.

17. Supplant Your Sugary Beverages With Sugar-Free or Sparkling Water

Sugary refreshments may conceivably be the unhealthiest thing you can drink.

They are stacked with fluid sugar, which has been connected to various diseases, including coronary illness, stoutness, and type 2 diabetes.

Likewise, your cerebrum doesn't enroll fluid calories a similar way it registers strong calories. This implies you don't make up for the calories you drink by eating any less.

One 17-ounce (500-ml) sugary soft drink may contain around 210 calories.

Have a go at supplanting your sugary refreshment with either a without sugar elective or basically pick still or shimmering water.

Doing so will shave off the additional calories and reduce your abundance of sugar and calorie admissions.

18. Avoid "Diet" Foods

Supposed "diet foods" can be very misleading.

They've normally had their fat substance reduced drastically and are frequently marked "sans fat," "low-fat," "fat-reduced," or "low-calorie."

Be that as it may, to make up for the lost flavor and surface that the fat gave, sugar and different fixings are frequently included.

In this way, many diet foods wind up containing more sugar and, at times, significantly a larger number of calories than their full-fat partners.

19. Get a Good Night's Sleep

The significance of good rest can't be exaggerated.

Lack of sleep upsets craving guidelines, regularly prompting expanded hunger, which brings about expanded calorie admission and weight gain.

Actually, individuals who rest excessively minimal will, in general, weigh essentially more than the individuals who get enough rest.

Being restless likewise, contrarily influences fixation, efficiency, athletic execution, glucose digestion, and immune capacity.

In addition, it expands your danger of a few diseases, including incendiary diseases and coronary illness.

Thusly, it is essential to attempt to get satisfactory measures of good-quality rest, ideally in one session.

20. Eat Fresh Berries Instead of Dried Ones

Berries are extremely healthy and pressed with supplements, fiber, and antioxidants.

Most assortments can be bought crisp, solidified, or dried.

Albeit various types are moderately healthy, the dried assortments are a significantly more thought wellspring of calories and sugar, since all the water has been evacuated.

A 3.5-ounce (100-gram) serving of crisp or solidified berries contains 32–35 calories, while 3.5 ounces of dried strawberries contain an incredible 396 calories.

The dried assortments are likewise regularly secured with sugar, further expanding the sugar content.

By settling on the crisp assortments, you will get a lot juicier tidbit that is lower in sugar and a ton lower in calories.

21. Eat Popcorn Instead of Chips

It might be amazing that popcorn is a whole grain that is stacked with supplements and fiber.

A 3.5-ounce (100-gram) serving of air-popped popcorn contains 387 calories and 15 grams of fiber, while a similar measure of chips contains 547 calories and just 4 grams of fiber.

Diets wealthy in whole grains have been connected to medical advantages, for example, a reduced danger of inflammation and coronary illness.

For healthy popcorn, take a stab at making your own popcorn at home (not microwave popcorn assortments) or buy air-popped popcorn.

Numerous business assortments set up their popcorn with fat, sugar, and salt, making it no more advantageous than potato chips.

22. Pick Healthy Oils

Lamentably, profoundly prepared seed and vegetable oils have become a family unit staple in the course of recent decades.

Models incorporate soybean, cottonseed, sunflower, and canola oils.

These oils are exceptionally handled and high in omega-6 unsaturated fats, however inadequate in omega-3s.

A high omega-6 to omega-3 proportion can prompt inflammation and has been connected to chronic diseases, for example, coronary illness, malignant growth, osteoporosis, and autoimmune diseases.

Swap these unhealthy oils for more beneficial other options, for example, additional virgin olive oil, avocado oil, or coconut oil.

23. Eat From Smaller Plates

Eating from an enormous plate can make your bit look littler while eating from a little plate can make it look greater.

Studies have upheld this and indicated that individuals would, in general, eat as much as 30% more when their food is served in a huge bowl or on an enormous plate.

Additionally, if you don't understand what you're eating more than expected, you won't repay by eating less at the

By eating from littler dinnerware, you can fool your mind into imagining that you're eating more, making yourself less inclined to overeat.

24. Get the Salad Dressing as an afterthought

Basically, arriving at the purpose of having the option to arrange a serving of mixed greens at an eatery is a great accomplishment for certain individuals.

Be that as it may, your endeavors ought not to end there. A few servings of mixed greens are covered in fatty dressings, which may make the plates of mixed greens considerably higher in calories than different things on the menu.

Requesting the dressing as an afterthought makes it significantly simpler to control the part size and along these lines, the calories that you expend.

25. Drink Your Coffee Black

Espresso, which is one of the most well-known refreshments on the planet, is healthy.

Actually, it is a significant wellspring of antioxidants and has been connected to numerous medical advantages, for example, a lower danger of diabetes, mental decrease, and liver sickness.

Be that as it may, numerous business assortments of espresso contain loads of extra fixings, for example, sugar, syrup, overwhelming cream, sugars, and milk. A considerable lot of these beverages are for all intents and purposes treats in a cup.

Drinking these assortments rapidly nullifies the entirety of espresso's medical advantages and rather includes loads of undesirable calories and sugar.

Rather, take a stab at drinking your espresso dark or simply including a modest quantity of milk or cream and abstain from improving it.

TIPS FOR SUCCESS

Your body is furnished with its own inner insurance component: the immune framework. It fends off colds, bug chomps, and significant disease, and endeavors to keep your body working appropriately. One of the symptoms of your immune framework kicking in is an expansion in inflammation. While this is a totally normal procedure, the issue lies when your body is in a steady condition of inflammation, known as "chronic inflammation." And when your body is doing combating inflammation of any sort, an anti-fiery diet can help assuage your manifestations and even lower the inflammation itself.

We addressed two dietitians to assemble this anti-provocative diet explainer: a manual for how this diet can assist you with bringing down the chronic inflammation that is the base of weight gain, skin issues, and stomach related problems.

Who would it be able to help?

An anti-fiery diet may fill in as a corresponding therapy for some conditions that become more terrible with chronic inflammation.

The accompanying conditions include inflammation:

- rheumatoid joint pain
- psoriasis
- asthma
- eosinophilic esophagitis
- Crohn's sickness
- colitis
- inflammatory inside infection
- lupus
- Hashimoto's sickness
- metabolic disorder

Metabolic disorder alludes to an assortment of conditions that will, in general, happen together, including type 2 diabetes, corpulence, hypertension, and cardiovascular infection.

Researchers accept that inflammation assumes a job in these. An anti-incendiary diet may, thusly, help improve the wellbeing of an individual with a metabolic disorder.

Eating a diet that is wealthy in antioxidants may likewise help reduce the danger of specific malignant growths.

Antioxidants assist evacuate with liberating radicals; however, what are free radicals? Discover here.

Foods to eat

An anti-incendiary diet should consolidate an assortment of foods that:

- are wealthy in supplements
- provide a scope of antioxidants
- contain energizing fats

Foods that may help oversee inflammation include:

- oily fish, for example, fish and salmon
- fruits, for example, blueberries, blackberries, strawberries, and fruits
- vegetables, including kale, spinach, and broccoli
- beans
- nuts and seeds
- olives and olive oil
- fiber
- raw or tolerably cooked vegetables
- legumes, for example, lentils
- spices, for example, ginger and turmeric
- probiotics and prebiotics
- tea
- some herbs

It merits recollecting that:

No single food will support an individual's wellbeing. It is imperative to remember an assortment of fortifying elements for the diet.

Crisp, straightforward fixings are ideal. Preparing can change the wholesome substance of foods.

Individuals should check the marks of premade foods. While cocoa can be a decent decision, for instance, the items that contain cocoa frequently likewise contain sugar and fat.

A beautiful plate will give a scope of antioxidants and different supplements.

Foods to avoid

Individuals who are following an anti-provocative diet ought to maintain a strategic distance from or limit their admission of:

- processed foods
- foods with included sugar or salt
- unhealthful oils
- processed carbs, which are available in white bread, white pasta, and many heated products
- processed nibble foods, for example, chips and wafers
- premade sweets, for example, treats, sweets, and frozen yogurt
- excess liquor
- In expansion, individuals may think that its valuable to confine their admission of the accompanying:

Gluten: Some individuals experience an incendiary response when they expend gluten. A without gluten diet can be prohibitive, and it isn't reasonable for everybody. Nonetheless, if an individual speculates that gluten is activating side effects, they may wish to consider dispensing with it for some time to check whether their manifestations improve.

Nightshades: Plants having a place with the nightshade family, for example, tomatoes, eggplants, peppers, and potatoes, appear to trigger flares in certain individuals with provocative diseases. There are constrained proof to affirm this impact, yet an individual can take a stab at cutting nightshades from the diet for 2–3 weeks to check whether their manifestations improve.

Sugars: There is some proof that a high carb diet, in any event, when the carbs are energizing, may advance inflammation in certain individuals. Nonetheless, some carb-rich foods, for example, sweet potatoes and whole grains, are great wellsprings of antioxidants and different supplements.

Could a vegetarian diet reduce inflammation?

A vegetarian diet might be one alternative for individuals hoping to reduce inflammation. Individuals who follow a vegetarian-based diet are probably going to have lower levels of different incendiary markers.

Anti-fiery diet tips

It very well may be trying to change to another method for eating, yet the accompanying tips may help:

- Pick up an assortment of organic products, vegetables, and invigorating snacks during the week after week shop.
- Gradually supplant cheap food meals with invigorating, custom made snacks.
- Replace pop and other sugary refreshments with still or shining mineral water.

Different tips include:

- Talking to social insurance proficient about enhancements, for example, cod liver oil or a multivitamin.
- Including a 30 minutes of moderate exercise into the day by day schedule.
- Practicing great rest cleanliness, as poor rest can decline inflammation.

An anti-incendiary diet may help reduce inflammation and improve the side effects of some basic wellbeing conditions, for example, rheumatoid joint pain.

There is no single anti-fiery diet, yet a diet that incorporates a lot of crisp products of the soil, whole grains, and energizing fats may help oversee inflammation.

Any individual who has a chronic well-being condition that includes inflammation ought to get some information about the best dietary choices for them.

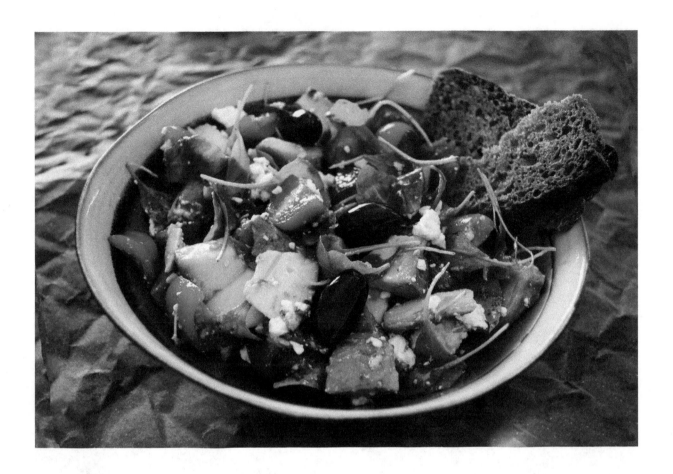

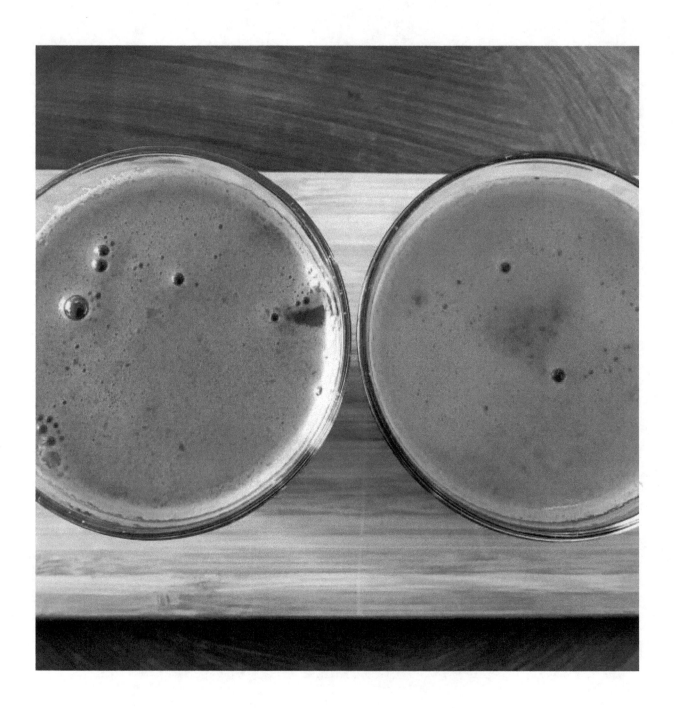

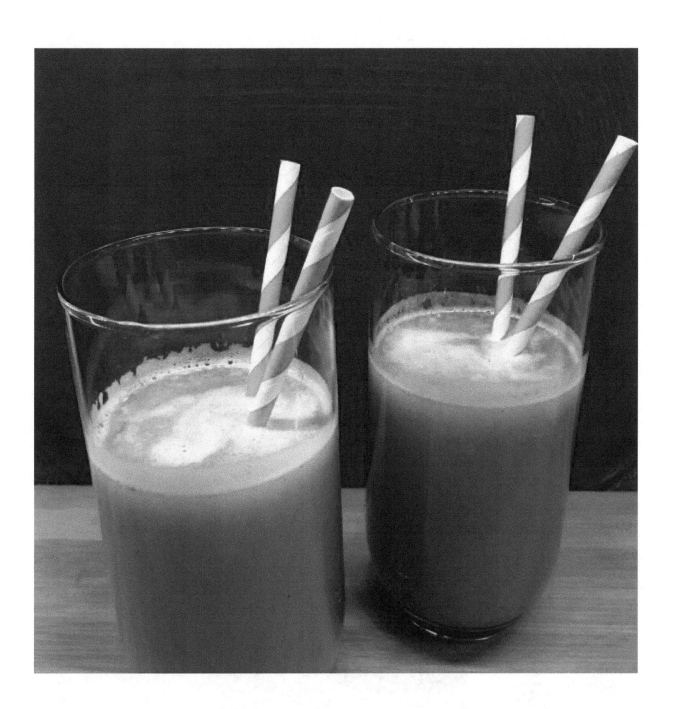

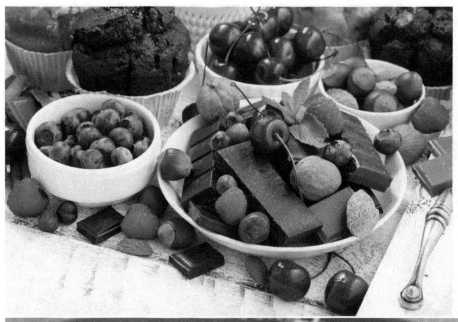

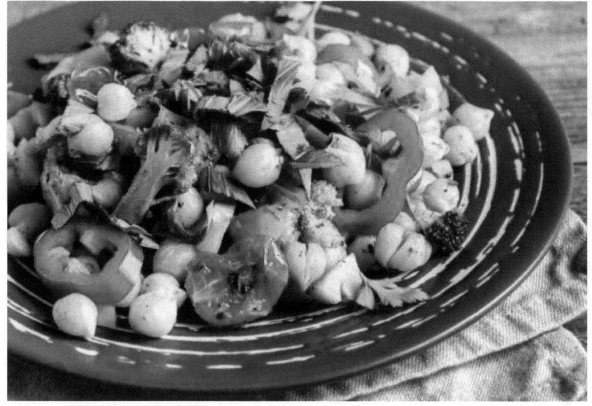